Also from Prentice Hall Press

The American Diabetes Association / The American Dietetic Association
Family Cookbook, Volume I (Revised Edition)
Family Cookbook, Volume II (Revised Edition)
Family Cookbook, Volume III (With Microwave Adaptations)
American Diabetes Association Holiday Cookbook
Betty Wedman, M.S., R.D.

American Diabetes Association.

Special Celebrations and Parties Cookbook

Betty Wedman, M.S., R.D.

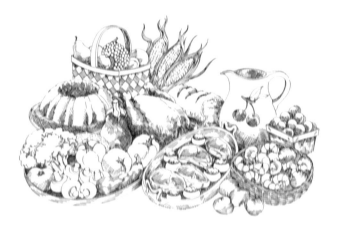

Prentice Hall Press

New York   London   Toronto   Sydney   Tokyo

Prentice Hall Press
15 Columbus Circle
New York, New York 10023

Copyright © 1989 by American Diabetes Association and Betty Wedman

PRENTICE HALL PRESS and colophon are registered
trademarks of Simon & Schuster, Inc.

Library of Congress Cataloging-in-Publication Data

Wedman, Betty.
    American Diabetes Association special celebrations and parties
cookbook / American Diabetes Association, Betty Wedman.
        p.   cm.
    Includes index.
    ISBN 0-13-004219-6 : $19.95
    1. Diabetes—Diet therapy—Recipes.   2. Entertaining.
I. American Diabetes Association.   II. Title.   III. Title: Special
celebrations and parties cookbook.
    RC662.   W362   1989
    641.5'6314—dc20   89-42674
                                                        CIP

Designed by Virginia Pope-Boehling
Manufactured in the United States of America

10 9 8 7 6 5 4 3 2 1

First Edition

To the people throughout the world who live with diabetes 365 days a year, 24 hours a day. Each one strives for "good" blood-glucose control in a less than well-controlled world full of temptations.

Daily activities are very food-oriented and it is hard to keep saying no. Now you can take your own food to a special celebration or party and feel confident that it fits into your diabetes meal plan.

Acknowledgments

I offer a special thank-you to my friends and associates who gave me the encouragement and support needed to complete this book and my doctoral research at the same time and to the American Diabetes Association (ADA) for allowing me to share these cooking and meal-planning tips for holidays and special celebrations. The ADA reviewers for this book were Madelyn L. Wheeler, M.S., R.D., C.D.E., and Louise E. Goggans, D.M.Sc., R.D. The introductory text was written by ADA Senior Editor Marcia Mazur. Many thanks to Susan Coughlin for her patience and dedication in getting this book published.

Contents

Foreword

*F*ood is health; food is life.

But food is more than that. Food is celebration. It's good times and good fellowship. It's parties, holidays, memories, and traditions. Food gathers family and welcomes friends. Food offers a gift to the guest, a present for the hostess. Food marks the births, marriages, and graduations of our lives and brings together the old and the young, the wanderer and the stay-at-home. Food expresses the joy of the moment, or marks our pleasure at the changing seasons.

Yet, for people with diabetes, food may also be a reminder of their disease, a taunt that tells them they are different, a constant hurdle, a continuing concern.

Today, however, those negative feelings can be a thing of the past. Recipes like those presented in the *American Diabetes Association Special Celebrations and Parties Cookbook*, have helped change the meaning of food for people with diabetes. Like its earlier companion, the *American Diabetes Association Holiday Cookbook*, this volume offers special-day recipes appropriate not only for people with diabetes but for everyone.

Whether it's a Thanksgiving Day feast, Fourth of July barbecue, Mother's Day brunch, or birthday bash, these recipes invite everyone to pull up a chair and enjoy.

This book also complements the three-volume Family Cookbook series coauthored by the American Diabetes Association and The American Dietetic Association. Recipes presented in all of these cookbooks are not only healthy but also delicious and satisfying. By taking into account the dietary needs of people with diabetes, they provide dishes everyone can eat, meals that bring people together. They break down the old barriers of special diets and special menus for individuals with diabetes.

Helping people with diabetes live healthy lives is what the American Diabetes Association (ADA) is all about. Today, diabetes affects some 11 million people in the United States, almost half of them still undiagnosed. And this chronic disease is on the rise. As the nation's largest voluntary health organization concerned with diabetes, the American Diabetes Association's mission is to prevent and cure diabetes and to improve the lives of all people affected by diabetes.

We do this through cookbooks like this one, and through our lively, easy-to-understand consumer magazine, *Diabetes Forecast*. Each monthly issue is packed with current information about diabetes and its control, as well as articles on diet and pages of recipes.

We also distribute a free quarterly newsletter with practical advice and helpful information on living with diabetes. In addition, we maintain a library of books, pamphlets, and brochures on all aspects of diabetes. This information is geared to people of all ages who have the disease and to those who care for and about them.

The American Diabetes Association also pursues its mission through generous funding of research that is making life better and healthier for the millions who have diabetes. Equally important, we support research that we hope will one day eliminate diabetes altogether, so future generations do not have to live with this serious disease.

The American Diabetes Association also works to help alert people who do not know they have diabetes. The sooner they are diagnosed, the sooner they can control the disease and help prevent possible long-term complications.

Our mission is carried on through ADA affiliates in fifty states and Puerto Rico and by dedicated men and women in ADA chapters in hundreds of communities throughout the United States. Together, the members of the American Diabetes Association work to bring a better life to people with diabetes and their families, wherever they live.

Membership in the American Diabetes Association puts you in contact with approximately 240,000 other people who have the same needs and are fighting the same enemy. Our local affiliates and chapters offer support groups, educational programs, counseling, and other services.

Information on ADA membership, programs and literature is available through our state affiliates, which are listed in the white pages of the telephone directory, or through the American Diabetes Association, Inc., Diabetes Information Service Center, 1660 Duke Street, Alexandria, Virginia 22314, 1-800-ADA-DISC. (In Virginia and the Washington, D.C., area, dial 703-549-1500.)

We hope you enjoy the *Special Celebrations and Parties Cookbook*. We wish you the joy of good food and the pleasure of good health. Bon appétit!

AMERICAN DIABETES ASSOCIATION

1

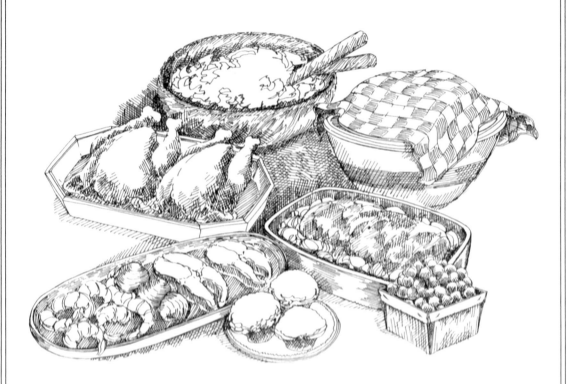

The Basics

*W*e all need good nutrition, and the principles of good nutrition are the same for all of us.

Nutritional Guidelines for Everyone

Here are current nutritional guidelines that combine information from government experts with recommendations from the American Diabetes Association (ADA) for people with both insulin-dependent (type I) and non-insulin-dependent (type II) diabetes. Their goal is to promote healthful eating for everyone.

1. *Eat a variety of foods.* To stay healthy, our bodies require up to fifty known nutrients. No single food contains them all. The wider the variety of foods we include in our diets, the less likely we'll be to develop either a deficiency or an excess of a single nutrient. Variety also reduces the likelihood of exposure to large amounts of contaminants in any single food, a growing concern in today's world.

To have variety in the daily diet, we have to choose foods from each of the major food groups: starches/breads, meats/meat substitutes, vegetables, fruits, milk/milk products, and fats. It's just as important to vary the foods within each food group.

2. *Maintain proper weight by controlling calories and exercising.* Calories are the basic units of measurement for the energy our bodies take in and use. When the food we eat provides more calories than we need, the body stores most of the unused calories as fat. We gain weight.

To lose one pound of body fat, we must cut 3,500 calories from our food intake. Cutting 500 calories a day from our diet will usually equal one pound of weight lost per week. It's easier to do that when we know where those calories are coming from.

The body gets its energy (calories) from four sources: protein, carbohydrate, fat, and alcohol. But those sources don't provide calories in equal numbers. Measure for measure, fat brings twice as many calories as other sources. To lose weight, it helps to cut down on foods of all kinds, but it's particularly good to cut down on fat. Alcohol is almost as high in calories as fat, and in fact, the body processes alcohol in much the same way as fat. Limiting alcohol intake is also helpful in losing weight.

Exercise of any kind will help use up calories, and that's particularly important for people with non-insulin-dependent diabetes, who are usually trying to lose weight.

Exercise also affects the insulin needs of people with insulin-dependent diabetes. For people on intensive insulin therapy or the insulin pump, it's best to get professional help to balance diet, insulin, and exercise to meet specific personal needs.

3. Limit fats and high-fat foods. The average American consumes 40 to 50 percent of his or her total calories in fat. Recently, the U.S. Surgeon General recommended that all adults reduce fat consumption to 30 percent of total calorie intake.

For people with diabetes, fatty foods pose several additional problems. Excess fat—particularly saturated fats (those that come from animal products as well as coconut and palm oils) and cholesterol—may contribute to atherosclerosis and heart disease. Since people with diabetes already carry a high risk for atherosclerosis and heart disease, limiting fats is particularly good advice. For individuals with non-insulin-dependent diabetes, the excess calories in fats make it hard to maintain proper weight—an important means of control for type II diabetes. Certain kinds of cancer may also be linked to fat intake.

We can cut fat intake by making informed food choices—reading labels will help—eating smaller portions, trimming fat before cooking, and cooking with low-fat methods. Since saturated fats are considered more harmful than polyunsaturated or monounsaturated fats, it's good to try to maintain the following ratio in your diet: less than 10 percent saturated fats, up to 10 percent polyunsaturated fats, and 10 to 15 percent monounsaturated fats. We can also decrease fat intake by eating more dried peas and beans, grain products, fruits, vegetables, low-fat dairy products, and low-fat meats.

4. Reduce cholesterol consumption. High levels of cholesterol, like fats, are one of the factors that contribute to atherosclerosis and heart disease. Cholesterol, a fat-like substance found in foods made with animal products, can clog arteries and prevent the flow of blood, a particular danger for the heart and brain.

Since the liver makes much of the cholesterol the body needs, it's a good idea to cut down the cholesterol consumed in foods. Total cholesterol intake should be no more than about 300 milligrams a day. Dietary cholesterol is found in all animal products, but is especially high in organ meats like liver and in egg yolks. One egg yolk contains about 270 milligrams of cholesterol.

The American Diabetes Association recommends very limited consumption of organ meats and no more than three egg yolks a week. Foods that come from plants—like corn oil—contain no cholesterol. They often contain fat, however. Labels that say "no cholesterol" do not mean the product has no fat.

5. Increase the use of unrefined carbohydrates and limit intake of refined carbohydrates. Gram for gram, all carbohydrates have the same number of calories. But different high-carbohydrate foods vary in their overall nutritional value.

Biochemically, carbohydrates are subdivided into three groups. The terms *sugar* and *simple carbohydrate* (e.g., glucose, fructose) are usually applied to *monosaccharides*, which have one sugar group per molecule, and to *disaccharides* (e.g., common table sugar) which have two sugar groups per molecule. The term *complex carbohydrate* usually refers to *polysaccharides*, which have many sugar groups per molecule.

Complex carbohydrates are found primarily in legumes (beans and peas), grain products, and starchy vegetables. Simple carbohydrates are found in fruit and milk. Each is an important source of many essential nutrients, such as vitamins, minerals, and fiber.

When carbohydrates are processed or "refined" into commercial sugar and other sweeteners, however, they are left with calories but very little else of nutritional value. That's why calories in simple carbohydrates are often called "empty" or "naked."

We should all eat less sugar and other refined carbohydrates. People with diabetes who have good blood-glucose control and acceptable weight may be able to have modest amounts of refined carbohydrates, as determined by their doctor or dietitian. Experts tell us to replace some of the fats in our diet with complex carbohydrates, bringing complex carbohydrates up to 55 to 60 percent of the total calories in our daily diet, if possible.

6. Reduce protein. Most Americans could stand to cut back their protein consumption. Because protein is found in many of the foods we eat daily—meat, poultry, fish, cheese, peanut butter—we tend to eat more than the ADA recommendation of about 0.8 grams per kilogram of body weight for adults. That comes to about 44 grams of protein daily for a 120-pound woman, 62 grams for a 170-pound man. (A 3-ounce serving of meat contains 21 grams of protein. A cup of milk contains 8 grams.)

A diet high in protein causes the kidneys to work hard, and too much protein seems to accelerate kidney damage, particularly in people with diabetes. Individuals with diabetes who have kidney disease, or are at risk for it, should have a doctor prescribe the exact amount of protein in their diet plan. Because pregnant women and growing children may need more than the minimum recommendation for protein, it is particularly important for these two groups to have a doctor determine their appropriate protein intake.

7. Increase consumption of fiber-rich foods. Fiber, or roughage, is the portion of plants that the human body cannot readily digest. Rich sources of dietary fiber include complex or unrefined carbohydrates, such as fresh vegetables and fruits, whole grains, beans, peas, and nuts. That means that whole-wheat bread is richer in fiber than white bread, brown rice higher in fiber than white rice.

For all of us, fiber is helpful in maintaining regularity. Scientists have also found that fiber may help the body handle carbohydrates. For people with non-insulin-dependent diabetes, scientists have found evidence that dietary fiber helps lower cholesterol and control blood-sugar levels. It's not yet clear whether fiber helps lower blood-sugar levels in those who are insulin-dependent.

8. Reduce sodium (salt) intake. Too much sodium, like saturated fat, may be associated with health problems, particularly high blood pressure, which can accelerate complications of diabetes.

The primary source of sodium in the American diet is table salt, which is about 40 percent sodium. (One teaspoon of table salt weighs 5 grams and has about 2,000 milligrams of sodium.) The American Diabetes Association recommends no more than 1,000 milligrams of sodium per 1,000 calories or no more than 3,000 milligrams of sodium a day.

We eat large amounts of sodium in convenience foods of all kinds. Foods that are salty to the taste—bacon or pickles, for example— may contain high levels of sodium. But taste alone is not always an accurate indicator of the sodium content of food. Commercial soups, peanut butter, and salad dressings are a few of the common foods that often have substantial amounts of sodium. It pays to read the label.

9. Use alcohol sparingly, if at all. We should all be aware of the dangers of too much alcohol. Besides affecting our mental control, alcohol is high in calories and has almost no nutritional value. For people trying to lose weight, cutting back on alcohol can help.

For people who have diabetes, alcohol poses a special problem. It can cause low blood sugar (hypoglycemia). It can also mask an insulin reaction, making people think the person with diabetes is drunk, instead of being in need of immediate attention.

The general rule: Anyone who drinks should do so in moderation at all times. One or two drinks a day seem to cause no harm to most adults. Pregnant women, however, should avoid alcohol to be on the safe side.

People with diabetes should consult a doctor or dietitian about alcohol consumption; there may be special restrictions concerning times for drinking and the kinds and amounts of alcoholic beverages consumed. Also, anyone with diabetes should always let a companion know that he/she has diabetes, so any lightheadedness will not be dismissed as just alcohol-related.

Tips for Healthy Eating

Here are some tips for following the nutritional guidelines in this cookbook that will help you put together a healthy diet for any member of your family. In any meal:

• Limit the caloric sweetener (table sugar, molasses, honey, syrup, etc.) in each recipe to 1 teaspoon or less per serving. Use substitute sweeteners like Equal® or Sweet 'n Low® whenever possible, or in combination with a limited amount of other sweeteners.

• Make sure no more than 30 percent of the calories come from fats of any kind, particularly saturated (animal) fats. To do that, substitute margarine (or better yet, diet margarine) for butter, low-fat yogurt for sour cream, skim or low-fat milk for whole milk, low-fat cheese for regular cheese, and so forth.

• Limit egg yolks in recipes to ½ yolk per serving because egg yolks are very high in cholesterol. You can sometimes eliminate yolks by using only the white part for a portion of the eggs; for example, try one yolk and three whites in a three-egg recipe. It's good to keep egg yolk consumption down to not more than three a week.

• Try to eliminate as much salt as possible from any recipe. This includes onion, garlic, or celery salt. (You can sometimes handle this by switching from onion, garlic, or celery salt to the powder or flake forms, using only half the original amount.) Use unsalted water for cooking vegetables, pasta, rice, and the like. Use homemade soup stocks or low-sodium broth or bouillon, rather than the saltier varieties. Use fresh, home-cooked vegetables or those canned with no added salt, rather than the regular canned varieties. The goal is to stay below 400 milligrams of sodium per exchange. The American Diabetes Association does not encourage the use of "lite salt" or other salt substitutes, unless advised for specific circumstances.

• You may include some wine or beer in a recipe because the alcohol evaporates during cooking, leaving only the wine or beer flavor.

Diet Management Tips

Here are some more tips that can help you to change the way you eat.

• Make changes in your diet gradually. Don't try to do everything all at once. It may take longer to accomplish your goals, but the changes you make will be permanent!

• Set short-term, realistic goals. If weight loss is your goal, try to lose two pounds in two weeks, not twenty pounds in a week. Walk two blocks at first, not two miles. Success will come more easily, and you'll feel good about yourself!

• Reward yourself. When you make your short-term goal, do something special for yourself. Go to a movie, buy a new shirt, read a book, visit a friend.

• Measure foods. It is important to eat the right serving sizes of food. You will need to learn how to estimate the amount of food you are served. You can do this by measuring all the food you eat for a week or so. Measure liquids with a measuring cup. Some solid foods (tuna, cottage cheese, canned fruits) can be measured with a measuring cup, too. Measuring spoons (teaspoon, tablespoon) are used for measuring smaller amounts such as oil, salad dressing, or peanut butter. A scale can be very useful to measure almost anything, especially meat, poultry, and fish. All food should be measured or weighed after cooking.

Some food you buy uncooked will weigh less after you cook it. This is true of most meats. Starches often swell in cooking, so a small amount of uncooked starch will become larger when cooked. The following table shows some of the changes:

Starch Group

Food	Uncooked	Cooked
Oatmeal	3 level Tbsp.	½ cup
Cream of Wheat	2 level Tbsp.	½ cup
Grits	3 level Tbsp.	½ cup
Rice	2 level Tbsp.	⅓ cup
Spaghetti	¼ cup	½ cup
Noodles	⅓ cup	½ cup
Macaroni	¼ cup	½ cup
Dried Beans	3 Tbsp.	⅓ cup
Dried Peas	3 Tbsp.	⅓ cup
Lentils	2 Tbsp.	⅓ cup

Meat Group

Food	Uncooked	Cooked
Hamburger	4 oz.	3 oz.
Chicken	1 small drumstick	1 oz.
	½ of a whole chicken breast	2 oz.

• Read food labels. When you see the word "dietetic" on a food label, it means that something has been changed or replaced. It may have less salt, less fat, or less sugar. It does not mean that the food is sugar-free or calorie-free. Some dietetic foods may be useful. Those that contain 20 calories or less per serving may be eaten up to three times a day as free foods.

• Know your sweeteners. Two types of sweeteners are on the market: those with calories and those without calories. Sweeteners with calories, such as fructose, sorbitol, and mannitol, when used in large amounts may cause cramping and diarrhea. Remember, these sweeteners do have calories that add up. Sweeteners without calories include saccharin and aspartame (Equal®, NutraSweet®) and may be used in moderation.

If you have insulin-dependent diabetes:

• Plan for sick days. Before you become ill with the flu or a cold, ask your doctor, dietitian, and nurse for a special sick day plan. It is important to:

• Take your usual insulin dose

• Test your blood glucose regularly and check your urine for ketones

• Try drinking small sips of regular soft drinks, sweetened tea, sweetened gelatin, popsicles, fruit juice, or sherbet, if you can't keep regular food down

• Drink lots of liquids

• Call your doctor immediately if you can't keep any food down

• Prepare for insulin reactions. If you have symptoms of low blood glucose, test your blood to find out your blood-glucose level. Be sure to carry something with you at all times to treat low blood glucose. You could carry glucose tablets or hard candy.

• Plan for exercise. You may need to make some changes in your meal plan or insulin dose when you begin an exercise program. Check with your dietitian or doctor about this. Be sure to carry with you some form of carbohydrate (such as dried fruit or glucose tablets) to treat low blood glucose.

Additional information on these topics is available from your dietitian or doctor.

What Is Diabetes?

Diabetes is a disorder characterized by the body's failure to handle glucose (sugar) properly. Glucose is the fuel that the body derives from food and then turns into energy. That means that food and nutrition play a big role in controlling diabetes.

Insulin—a hormone produced in the pancreas—helps the glucose that is derived from foods enter the body's cells, where it is used. If the body produces no insulin or is unable to use its insulin properly, the result is high levels of glucose in the blood. High blood glucose can cause immediate problems, such as fatigue, excessive hunger, thirst, and frequent urination. It can also cause more serious long-term complications involving the kidneys, nerves, eyes, and blood circulation. Diabetes can also sometimes figure in heart disease and stroke.

There are two major forms of diabetes: insulin-dependent (type I) and non-insulin-dependent (type II).

Insulin-dependent diabetes. About 10 percent of the people in the United States

with diabetes are insulin-dependent (type I). This form of the disease usually appears in childhood, and almost always before age thirty. People who are insulin-dependent produce essentially no insulin and need daily injections of insulin to survive. After an injection, the insulin user must eat appropriate amounts of the right foods at the right times for the insulin to work on. The goal is to achieve and maintain a near-normal blood-glucose level.

This is quite a balancing act, because food is not the only factor that affects blood-glucose levels. Exercise, for instance, generally lowers blood glucose, and stress (whether emotional or physical) can raise it.

Non-insulin-dependent diabetes. People with this kind of diabetes do produce some insulin in their bodies. In fact, they may have a normal or even higher-than-normal amount; however, for various reasons, their insulin is not as effective as it should be. Often, this is largely due to excess body fat, which is common in people with type II diabetes. Non-insulin-dependent diabetes usually develops after age forty.

About 90 percent of people with diabetes have type II. About 80 percent of individuals with non-insulin-dependent diabetes are overweight at the time of diagnosis. For them, dieting often brings a remarkable improvement. Weight loss, followed by weight maintenance, is a major goal for overweight people with type II diabetes.

Some people with type II diabetes take pills to help control their blood glucose when weight loss and exercise programs do not do the job. This medication is not insulin, but it helps the body to use its own insulin more effectively. Some people with type II diabetes also receive insulin. People treated with insulin, and some who take pills, need to eat food in prescribed amounts at specific times.

Nutritional Guidelines for People with Diabetes

No matter what kind of diabetes you have, the following are goals of diet therapy:

• Provide adequate nutrition for normal growth and development at all stages of life.

• Maintain blood glucose at as close to normal levels as possible and maintain blood fats at optimal levels.

• Achieve and/or maintain a body weight appropriate for your height and age.

• Improve overall health through good nutrition.

To achieve these goals, the American Diabetes Association recommends the following general guidelines:

• Pay particular attention to your calories. Excess calories cause high blood-glucose levels and obesity.

• Limit your intake of refined carbohydrates (all kinds of sugars like table sugar, honey, molasses, corn sugar, syrup). In addition to being low in vitamins and other nutrients, these sugary foods cause a rapid and high rise in blood-glucose levels.

Does this guideline mean you can never have refined sugars? No. Today, there is a somewhat more liberal attitude toward use of refined carbohydrates in the diabetic diet. And, in fact, the recipes in the *Special Celebrations and Parties Cookbook* have slightly more sugar than found in recipes in previous American Diabetes Association cookbooks. (See "About These Recipes" on page 14.) Keep in mind, though, that the amount of refined carbohydrates appropriate for your diet depends on you—specifically on *your* blood-glucose control, *your* levels of blood fats, *your* weight and other factors.

The right amount of sugar for your diet can only be determined with advice from your doctor or dietitian. Be sure to check with your health-care team on how to work refined carbohydrates into your meal plan safely.

• Work with a dietitian familiar with diabetes to develop your personal meal plan.

Many dietitians recommend that you develop a meal plan based on the *Exchange Lists for Meal Planning*, a publication of the American Diabetes Association and The American Dietetic Association. (See page 217.)

The Exchange Lists

Eating the correct foods in the right proportions is one of the most important ways of controlling both insulin-dependent (type I) and non-insulin-dependent (type II) diabetes. But eating the right amount of the right foods at every meal, snack, party, or banquet can be difficult, not to mention downright dreary.

That is why the American Diabetes Association and The American Dietetic Association put together the *Exchange Lists for Meal Planning*, a way to maintain the diet yet add variety and sparkle to menus (see page 217).

Because foods vary in their carbohydrate, protein, fat, and calorie content, foods have been divided into six main lists. Two of the lists—meat and milk—have three sublists. Every food on each list—in the portion stated—has about the same amount of carbohydrate, protein, fat, and calories as every other item on the list. That means the stated amount of any item on the list can be exchanged for the stated portion of any other item on the same list.

The six exchange lists include

starch/bread	fruit
meat/meat substitutes	milk
lean	skim
medium-fat	low-fat
high-fat	whole
vegetable	fat

One choice in a list may call for a larger quantity of food than another item from the same list. Because foods vary in their nutritional composition, portions of different foods must also vary in order to bring nutrient values as close as possible to each other.

Also, foods on the exchange lists that are high in fiber (3 grams or more of fiber per exchange) are footnoted. These foods make particularly good choices because high-fiber foods are important in the diet.

Foods that are high in sodium (400 milligrams or more of sodium per exchange) are also noted. The American Diabetes Association recommends no more than 1,000 milligrams of sodium per 1,000 calories or not more than 3,000 milligrams of sodium per day.

The current exchange lists also emphasize carbohydrates and downplay meats, which contain saturated fats.

Using the Exchange Lists

To use the exchange lists, you and your dietitian must first figure the number of calories, carbohydrates, protein, fats, fiber, and sodium your body needs each day for your particular age and lifestyle. Your dietitian can then help you translate those nutrients into the kind and number of food selections (or exchanges) you should eat at each meal and snack. That's your personal meal plan.

Armed with this meal plan, you can select from the choice of items within each exchange list and still keep the appropriate number of nutrients. This allows for a nutritious diet composed of a variety of foods that can help keep the sparkle in your menu.

Free foods. The exchange lists also have free foods. These are foods or drinks that contain less than 20 calories per serving. Enjoy as much as you want of those that have no serving size specified. You can eat two or three servings per day of those items that have a specific serving size, but not all at one time.

Many condiments and seasonings are also classified as free foods. The exchange lists specify condiments like catsup, horseradish, mustard, taco sauce, as well as herbs and seasonings, and the like. (Note:

You may still have to watch serving size, though.) By using condiments and seasonings, you can break away from humdrum flavors, introduce new tastes, and still maintain your diet plan. Although you can be liberal in using spices, herbs, and some condiments, watch out for sodium that might be in a condiment like pickles.

Combination foods. You might wonder how you handle foods composed of more than one item, for example, a casserole or a pudding. The exchange lists also provide exchange values for some typical combinations of foods. Your dietitian can be a big help in teaching you to calculate exchange values for combination foods yourself. Cookbooks like this one are also a great help because they have already calculated exchanges for you.

If you have recipes that you enjoy and use often, you may wish to convert them to exchanges. The following steps will help.

1. List all the ingredients in the recipe and their amounts.

2. Identify the exchange group and record the number of exchanges in each ingredient.

3. Total each exchange group.

4. Divide the total number of exchanges for each group by the number of servings in the recipe and round off to the nearest ½ exchange. Anything less than ½ need not be counted.

Here's an example, using a recipe for macaroni and cheese that yields 4 ½-cup servings.

Step 1. List ingredients	Step 2. Identify Exchange Groups
2 cups cooked macaroni	4 starches/breads
¼ cup onion, chopped	½ vegetable (free)
½ teaspoon salt	Free
Dash Tabasco sauce	Free
¼ cup skim milk	¼ skim milk
1 cup (4 ounces) skim or part-skim cheese	4 medium-fat meats

Step 3. Total Exchange Groups	Step 4. Divide by Number of Servings
4 starches/breads	by 4 = 1 starch/bread
¼ skim milk	by 4 = negligible
4 medium-fat meats	by 4 = 1 medium-fat meat

Result:
One serving of macaroni and cheese equals 1 starch/bread exchange and 1 medium-fat meat exchange.

Foods for occasional use. Even if you've got diabetes, you can occasionally have small portions of foods with higher than usual sugar or fat content—as long as you keep your blood glucose under control. That's why the exchange lists include foods for occasional use—treats like angel food cake, cookies, even ice cream. The important thing to remember is that these foods must be carefully worked into your meal plan. Check them with your doctor or dietitian.

Recipes do not list the amount of sugar per serving, so the cook must calculate the amount before considering whether to make a recipe. When calculating the amount of sugar in a recipe, be sure to include the following ingredients, which are different forms of sugar: corn syrup, honey, molasses, maple syrup, and pancake syrup.

Let's take a recipe and calculate how much sugar is in one serving.

Angel Food Cake

10 egg whites
1¼ teaspoons cream of tartar
¼ teaspoon salt
1 teaspoon vanilla extract
½ teaspoon almond extract
1¼ cups sugar
1 cup cake flour

The recipe serves eight and calls for 1¼ cups of sugar. One cup equals 16 tablespoons. One-fourth cup equals 4 tablespoons. That means there are 20 tablespoons of sugar in the recipe. Each tablespoon of sugar equals 3 teaspoons. So, 20 × 3 = 60 teaspoons of sugar in the total recipe for angel food cake (serves 8).

To calculate the amount of sugar per serving, divide 60 teaspoons by 8. That means each serving of angel food cake equals 7½ teaspoons of sugar.

If the slices of angel food cake are made smaller and 12 servings are cut, one serving of angel food cake now equals 5 teaspoons of sugar (60 teaspoons divided by 12). The high sugar content tells you why angel food cake is used only as a special treat on the diabetes meal plan.

About These Recipes

The recipes in this cookbook were specially developed and field-tested with an eye to helping anyone follow the nutritional guidelines for people with diabetes, most of which are recommended for all Americans interested in sound nutrition. In general, the recipes are:

▪ Reduced in total fat as well as saturated (animal) fat (no more than 2 fat exchanges per serving)

▪ Reduced in cholesterol (no more than 300 milligrams per serving)

▪ Limited to ½ egg per serving in recipes calling for eggs

▪ Limited in salt and sodium-rich ingredients (recipes with 400 milligrams or more of sodium per serving are flagged)

▪ Limited to 1 teaspoon or less of sugar, honey, molasses, or other caloric sweeteners per serving when a recipe includes these ingredients. Some recipes contain moderate amounts of these sweeteners (more than 1 teaspoon and less than 1 tablespoon per serving). Since these recipes also contain less than 300 calories per serving, they may be appropriate for occasional use; however, they should be carefully worked into the meal plan with advice from a doctor or dietitian. These recipes are identified with the notation "For Occasional Use Only."

In addition, each recipe provides a nutrient analysis per serving that includes

Calories
Protein
Carbohydrate
Fat
Sodium
Potassium
Cholesterol

Food exchange values per serving are provided for each recipe. The exchanges were calculated using the *Exchange Lists for Meal Planning*, published by the American Diabetes Association and The American Dietetic Association (see page 217).

Unless noted otherwise, the nutrient analysis for recipes using chicken is calculated for chicken without skin. For recipes using chicken or beef broth, the regular canned variety was used; you can reduce the amount of sodium per serving by substituting homemade or low-sodium broth. You can reduce the sodium in recipes calling for canned beans by substituting fresh beans. For recipes calling for a variable amount of one ingredient—for example, 2½ to 3 cups of flour—the nutrient analysis was calculated using the midpoint amount (2¾ cups in our example). For recipes using a marinade, the nutrient analysis assumes that one-half of the marinade is absorbed.

2

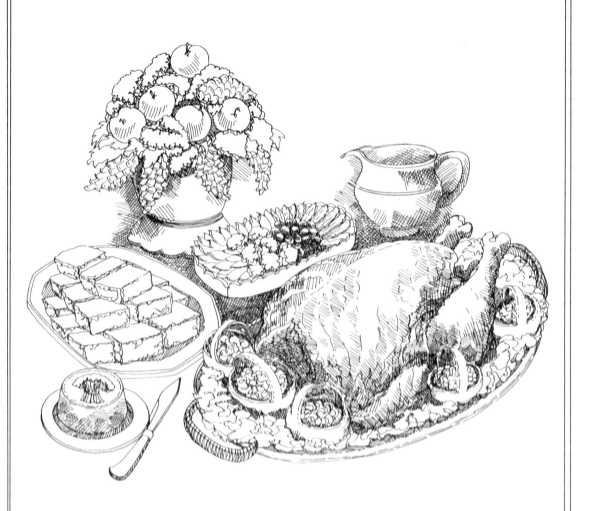

Menus

New Year's Day

Chicken with Raspberry Sauce
Parsnips and Snow Peas
Carrot and Grape Salad
Oatmeal Muffins
Cheesecake

Valentine's Day

Creamed Scallops and Lobster
on Noodles
Green Beans
Basil and Cheese Bread Sticks
Margarine
Apple and Cheese Pizza

Presidents' Day

Pork Chops with Red Cabbage
and Apples
Noodles
Vegetable Salad
Pear Muffins
Sponge Roll with Strawberry Filling

Purim

Chicken with Fruit and Cashews
Baby Carrots à la Mint
Hamantaschen

St. Patrick's Day

Watercress Soup
Fillet of Sole Florentine
Parsnips and Snow Peas
Irish Soda Bread
Apple Raisin Snack Cake

Easter

Minted Lamb Roast with Apples
Baked Potato
Margarine
Mixed Vegetables
Crisp Lettuce Salad and Caesar
Salad Dressing
Hot Cross Bun

Easter Supper

Italian Easter Pie
Fruit and Vegetable Tray
Kulich

Passover

Purée of Broccoli Soup
Baked Chicken with Matzo Stuffing
Two Bean–Orange Salad
Pickled Beets
Passover Popovers
Banana Passover Cake

Mother's Day Brunch

Orange French Toast
Shrimp-Crab-Pasta Salad
Tossed Salad and Italian Dressing
Herbed Popover

Mother's Day Dinner

(Easy enough for every family
member to contribute to making this
a special meal for Mother)

Deviled Eggs
Chicken Breasts Scallopini
Bran Cereal Muffins
Margarine
Date Bars

Memorial Day

Seafood Kabob Appetizers
Pork Tenderloin Dijon on Fettuccine
Zucchini and Carrots
Strawberry Bread
Margarine
Peanut Butter Cookies

Father's Day

South Atlantic Crab Bites
Brown Rice Chicken Salad
Hearty Baked Beans
Feta Cheese Casserole Bread
Nectarine Waldorf Dessert

Special Father's Day Dinner

Bouillabaisse
Cardamom Pot Roast
Potatoes and Carrots
Bran Buttermilk Biscuit
Margarine
Pineapple Upside-Down Cake

Fourth of July Barbecue

Sugar-free Lemonade
Grilled Prawns
Honey-Basted Cornish Hens
Red Potatoes in Parchment
Vegetable Salad
Blueberry Mousse

Fourth of July Salad Buffet

Orange and Blue Smoothee
Scallops Pasta Salad
Beet Salad with Orange Dressing
Sweet and Sour Cucumbers
Red, White, and Blue Salad
Corn-Oatmeal Muffin
Blueberry Kugel

Other Fourth of July Choices

Chicken with Raspberry Sauce
Blueberry Torte Dessert

Labor Day

Gazpacho
Grapefruit Chicken and Vegetables
Corn-Potato Hash
Pea Salad
Pickled Pears
Pickled Watermelon Rind
Italian Plum Muffins
Frozen Fruit Delight

Rosh Hashanah

Beef Stew with Acorn Squash
or
Cornish Hen with Wild Rice Stuffing
or
Baked Fish with Tomato-Pepper Sauce
Noodle Kugel with Vegetables
Apple Cake
or
Baked Apples

Yom Kippur

Gefilte Fish Loaf
Veal and Bean Cholent
Red Potatoes in Parchment
Pea Salad
Sweet-and-Sour Cucumbers
Pear-Nut Bread
Apple-Raisin Snack Cake

Sukkoth

Pineapple-Grapefruit-Avocado Salad
Stuffed Cabbage
Wild Rice
Green Bean and Red Pepper Salad
or
Carrot and Grape Salad
Sponge Cake

Halloween Party for Young People

Cheesy Snack Balls
Peanut Butter Popcorn
Fruit Leather
Oatmeal Raisin Muffins
Pumpkin Pudding Cake

Halloween Party for Adults

Medley Vegetable Soup
Pumpkin Bran Muffins
Snappy Pumpkin Mousse

Intimate Thanksgiving Feast

Eggplant Caviar with Raw Vegetables
Roast Turkey
Wild Rice
Green Beans and Mushrooms
Almondine
Cranberry Muffin

Thanksgiving Dinner

Smoked Salmon Dip
Apple-Pecan Salad
Roast Turkey
Zucchini Spoonbread
Baby Carrots à la Mint
Mincemeat-Oatmeal Muffin
Pumpkin Pie

Thanksgiving Supper

Turkey-Chestnut Salad
Marinated Mushrooms
Oatmeal-Pumpkin Bread
Swedish Hazelnut Squares

Other Choices for Thanksgiving

Baked Apples and Mincemeat
Pumpkin-Bran Muffins
Pumpkin Cheesecake
Apple-Mincemeat Pie
Pumpkin-Mincemeat Pie
Gingerbread Cookies
Brandied Pear Fruitcake

Christmas Brunch

Mincemeat Swirls
Cardamom Christmas Ring
Two Bean–Orange Salad
Fresh Fruit Cup

Christmas Dinner

Citrus Fizz Punch
Watercress, Beet, and Orange Salad
Roast Turkey
Glazed Sweet Potatoes
Spiced Cauliflower
Greek Christmas Loaf
Individual Fruitcake

Other Christmas Favorites

Mincemeat Cake

Pear-Nut Bread

Mincemeat-Banana Bread

Peanut Butter Cookies

Mincemeat Cookies

Black Walnut Squares

Molasses Cookies

Hanukkah

Lentil-Potato Patties

Baked Beef Brisket

or

Rainbow Trout with Saffron

Rice Stuffing

Eggplant-Tomato Salad

Sourdough Rye Bread

Refrigerator Spice Cookies

Graduation Buffet

Pizza Chicken

Chili Pie

Cheese Pizza Bread

Corn-Oatmeal Muffins

Zucchini Casserole

Apple-Raisin Snack Cake

Teen Birthday Party

Impossible Pizza Pie

Raw Vegetable Nibbles

Molasses Cookies

Birthday Buffet

Bon Bon Chicken

Paella

Broccoli Spears

Two Bean–Orange Salad

Brownies

3

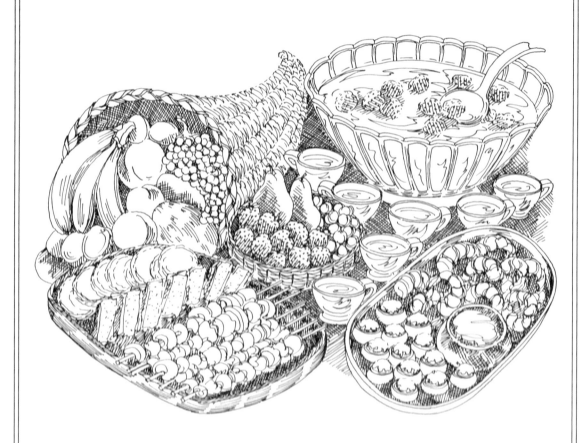

Appetizers and Beverages

Bon Bon Chicken

1 pound chicken wings
1 tablespoon sesame or
  vegetable oil
1 tablespoon toasted sesame
  seeds
1 green onion, finely chopped
1 packet sugar substitute
2 tablespoons soy sauce
¼ teaspoon cayenne pepper

Yield: 10 appetizer servings of
6 pieces.

Food Exchanges: 3 lean meats +
1 fat

Cut chicken wings into sections. Cook in boiling water until tender. Cool thoroughly. Mix remaining ingredients in a bowl and pour over chicken wings. Toss to coat chicken. Chill until ready to serve. Arrange on platter. Reheat or serve cold.

Calories per serving	217
Protein	19 g
Carbohydrate	0
Fat	15 g
Sodium	228 mg
Potassium	135 mg
Cholesterol	58 mg

Marinated Mushrooms

1 pound fresh mushrooms
½ cup lemon juice or vinegar
2 cloves garlic, minced
⅓ cup vegetable oil
2 teaspoons dried oregano
  leaves
1 teaspoon dried thyme leaves

Yield: 8 servings of 5
mushrooms

Food Exchange: 1 fat

Wash mushrooms and cut lengthwise through stem and top if they are large. Combine remaining ingredients and pour over mushrooms. Marinate for several hours or overnight in refrigerator.

Calories per serving	55
Protein	0.5 g
Carbohydrate	2 g
Fat	5 g
Sodium	3 mg
Potassium	96 mg
Cholesterol	0

Italian Calzone

1 tablespoon active dry yeast

1 cup warm water

4 cups all-purpose flour

½ teaspoon salt

1 teaspoon black pepper

2 eggs

¼ cup vegetable oil

¼ pound mozzarella cheese, thinly sliced

¼ pound prosciutto ham, thinly sliced

¼ pound capocollo ham, thinly sliced

¼ pound salami, thinly sliced

1½ pounds ricotta cheese

3 eggs

Cornmeal

Yield: 20 appetizer servings (or 10 lunch or brunch servings)

Food Exchanges: 2 medium-fat meats + 1 starch/bread

Make the dough by dissolving the yeast in water. Combine 2 cups of the flour, salt, pepper, 2 eggs, and oil in a mixing bowl. Beat to blend. Add yeast mixture and 1 cup flour to make kneadable dough. Pour dough on a floured surface using remaining cup of flour. Knead until smooth and elastic. Place in an oiled bowl and let rise in a warm place until doubled in bulk, about 1 hour.

Cut mozzarella, prosciutto, capocollo, and salami into thin, small pieces. Add to ricotta and mix to blend well. Add 3 eggs and beat thoroughly. Set aside.

After dough has doubled in size, divide in half. Roll each half into a large rectangle, about ½ inch thick. Spread half of filling over half of dough. Fold dough over and seal edges. Place on a baking sheet that has been covered with cornmeal. Repeat with other half of dough. Place in a 375-degree oven for 30 minutes or until crust is golden brown.

Calories per serving	251
Protein	14 g
Carbohydrate	19 g
Fat	13 g
Sodium	377 mg
Potassium	146 mg
Cholesterol	101 mg

Sautéed Shrimp Parmesan

½ *pound fresh or frozen*
shrimp
1 teaspoon margarine
1 clove garlic, minced
1 tablespoon grated Parmesan
cheese
1 tablespoon chopped fresh
parsley

Shell shrimp. Melt margarine in skillet. Add garlic and shrimp. Sauté for 3 to 4 minutes or just until shrimp are pink. Sprinkle on Parmesan cheese and parsley. Serve over rice.*

Calories per serving	62
Protein	12 g
Carbohydrates	0
Fat	1 g
Sodium	138 mg
Potassium	146 mg
Cholesterol	52 mg

Yield: 4 servings of 4 shrimp

Food Exchange: 1 lean meat

* *Rice is not included in the nutrient analysis for this recipe. One-third cup of cooked rice equals 1 starch/bread exchange.*

Seafood Kabob Appetizers

4 ounces fresh or frozen
shrimp
4 ounces scallops
8 cherry tomatoes
8 celery chunks
2 tablespoons low-calorie
Italian salad dressing

Remove shells from shrimp. Thread onto 4 skewers alternately with scallops, tomatoes, and celery. Brush with salad dressing. Broil for 3 to 4 minutes, turning frequently, until shrimp are pink.

Calories per serving	66
Protein	12 g
Carbohydrate	1 g
Fat	1 g
Sodium	145 mg
Potassium	263 mg
Cholesterol	16 mg

Yield: 4 servings

Food Exchange: 1 lean meat

South Atlantic Crab Bites

1 pound cooked crabmeat
½ cup cracker crumbs or bread
  crumbs
1 egg
¼ cup mayonnaise
1½ teaspoons prepared
  mustard
⅛ teaspoon ground cayenne
  pepper
2 tablespoons vegetable oil

Yield: 16 servings of 1 crab
cake

Food Exchange: 1 medium-fat
meat

Remove any cartilage from crabmeat. Add cracker crumbs, mustard, egg, mayonnaise, and pepper. Mix thoroughly. Divide into 16 small cakes. Pour oil in a no-stick skillet and add crab cakes. Cook over medium heat until browned, about 3 minutes on each side.

Calories per serving	74
Protein	4 g
Carbohydrate	2 g
Fat	5 g
Sodium	50 mg
Potassium	67 mg
Cholesterol	22 mg

Baked Sea Trout Fingers

1 pound sea trout fillets
2 egg whites
⅓ cup unsalted cashews
4 tablespoons grated Parmesan
  cheese
½ cup cornflakes

Cut fillets into strips. Beat egg whites until foamy. Combine cashews, Parmesan cheese, and cornflakes in a blender. Grind until fine. Empty into a shallow dish. Roll each fillet in egg and then into crumb mixture. Place on a lightly oiled baking sheet. Bake in a 400-degree oven for 5 minutes. Broil for 2 minutes until crisp.

Calories per serving	111
Protein	12 g
Carbohydrate	7 g
Fat	4 g
Sodium	166 mg
Potassium	284 mg
Cholesterol	48 mg

Yield: 8 1-strip servings

Food Exchanges: 2 lean meats

Grilled Prawns

*1 pound large shrimp or
    prawns, shelled*
8 mushrooms
1 teaspoon prepared mustard
½ teaspoon ground rosemary
¼ cup apple juice

Split prawns almost in half down the back. Press flat. Combine prawns and mushrooms in a bowl. Add remaining ingredients. Marinate for 4 hours or overnight. Alternate prawns and mushrooms on skewers. Grill over hot coals or broil 5 inches from heat. Turn frequently to cook all sides.

Calories per serving	107
Protein	22 g
Carbohydrate	2 g
Fat	1 g
Sodium	226 mg
Potassium	345 mg
Cholesterol	46 mg

Yield: 4 servings of 2 prawns

Food Exchanges: 3 lean meats

Smoked Salmon Dip

¼ pound smoked salmon
1½ cups low-fat cottage cheese
*1 to 2 tablespoons skim milk,
    if necessary*
2 tablespoons horseradish

Flake salmon with fork. Purée cottage cheese in blender (using skim milk, if necessary). Combine salmon, cottage cheese, and horseradish in a bowl. Cover and refrigerate for 3 hours or overnight to blend flavors. Serve with crackers or raw vegetables.

Calories per serving	51
Protein	8 g
Carbohydrate	2 g
Fat	1 g
Sodium	801 mg
Potassium	974 mg
Cholesterol	42 mg

Yield: 8 ¼-cup servings or 2 cups

Food Exchange: 1 lean meat

Note: This recipe contains 400 milligrams or more of sodium per serving.

Eggplant Caviar

*1 large eggplant (about 1
pound)*
1 tablespoon olive oil
1 clove garlic, minced
3 green onions, chopped
2 tablespoons lemon juice
*¼ teaspoon ground white
pepper*
*2 tablespoons toasted sesame
seeds*
*2 tablespoons minced fresh
parsley*
1 teaspoon salt (optional)
Capers

Yield: 6 ¼-cup servings

Food Exchanges: 1 vegetable +
½ fat

Peel eggplant. Cut into cubes and steam until tender. Sauté in a skillet with oil, garlic, and onions until all moisture has evaporated. Purée in a food processor or blender until smooth. Beat in remaining ingredients, except capers. Pour into serving bowl. Top with capers just before serving. Serve warm or cold on toast points, crackers, or vegetable slices.

Calories per serving	39
Protein	1 g
Carbohydrate	3 g
Fat	3 g
Sodium (no salt added)	1 mg
Potassium	86 mg
Cholesterol	0

Salsa

4 fresh ripe tomatoes, finely
  chopped
1 small onion, chopped
1 jalapeño pepper, stem and
  seeds removed
6 sprigs fresh cilantro or
  coriander
3 sprigs fresh parsley
1 16-ounce can tomato sauce
1 packet sugar substitute
1 tablespoon vegetable oil
1 tablespoon red wine vinegar

Yield: 5 ½-cup servings

Food Exchange: 1½ vegetables

Combine tomatoes and onion in bowl. Chop pepper, cilantro, and parsley. Purée all ingredients in a food processor or blender. Heat, if desired, to blend flavors by simmering over medium flame for 15 minutes. Cool. Serve over scrambled eggs, hamburgers, fish, or with chips.

Calories per serving	43
Protein	1 g
Carbohydrate	7 g
Fat	1.5 g
Sodium	265 mg
Potassium	318 mg
Cholesterol	0

Orange Peach Frosty

1 cup orange juice
2 tablespoons lime juice
1 cup sliced fresh or frozen
  peaches
Crushed ice
Fresh mint leaves

Yield: 4 ½-cup servings

Food Exchange: 1 fruit

Combine all ingredients in a blender. Purée until smooth. Serve immediately. Garnish with fresh mint leaves.

Calories per serving	49
Protein	0
Carbohydrate	13 g
Fat	0
Sodium	0
Potassium	214 mg
Cholesterol	0

Orange and Blue Smoothee

1 pint fresh or frozen
  blueberries
¼ cup orange juice
2 packets sugar substitute
1 cup plain low-fat yogurt
Strawberries

Prepare blueberry purée by cooking blueberries and orange juice together until skins pop, about 3 minutes. Add sugar substitute when cool. Combine ¼ cup yogurt and ¼ cup blueberry purée in a blender with crushed ice. Garnish with strawberry.

Calories per serving	84
Protein	3 g
Carbohydrate	16 g
Fat	1 g
Sodium	45 mg
Potassium	227 mg
Cholesterol	3.5 mg

Yield: 4 ½-cup servings

Food Exchange: 1 fruit

Citrus Fizz Punch

1 6-ounce can frozen grapefruit
  juice concentrate
1 6-ounce can frozen orange
  juice concentrate
¼ cup lemon juice
3 cups water
24 ounces sugar-free 7UP® or
  ginger ale
Ice cubes

Defrost grapefruit and orange juice concentrates. Mix in lemon juice and water. Pour into punch bowl. Add 7UP® and ice.

Calories per serving	41
Protein	0.5 g
Carbohydrate	10 g
Fat	0
Sodium	1 mg
Potassium	157 mg
Cholesterol	0

Yield: 16 ½-cup servings

Food Exchange: ½ fruit

Peach Fizz

1 ripe peach
Club soda or sugar-free 7UP®
Strawberry

Peel, pit, and slice peach. Purée in a food processor or blender until smooth. Pour purée into a champagne glass and fill with club soda. Top with fresh strawberry.

Calories per serving	57
Protein	0.9 g
Carbohydrate	14.7 g
Fat	0.1 g

Yield: 1 ½-cup serving

Sodium	0
Potassium	260 mg

Food Exchange: 1 fruit Cholesterol 0

Melon Shake

1½ cups cantaloupe cubes
1⅓ cups skim milk
½ teaspoon coconut extract
3 to 4 packets sugar substitute
Ice cubes

Combine all ingredients in a blender. Purée until smooth.

Calories per serving	64
Protein	4 g
Carbohydrate	13 g
Fat	0

Yield: 4 ½-cup servings

Sodium	51 mg
Potassium	445 mg

Food Exchange: 1 fruit Cholesterol 1 mg

Apricot Mint Julep

2 ripe fresh apricots
1 teaspoon lime juice
½ packet sugar substitute
2 fresh mint leaves
Ice cubes

Peel, pit, and slice apricots. Purée in a food processor or blender with lime juice, sugar substitute, and 1 mint leaf. Add 2 ice cubes or crushed ice. Process on and off to blend. Pour into serving glass. Garnish with mint leaf.

Calories per serving	34
Protein	0
Carbohydrate	8 g
Fat	0
Sodium	0
Potassium	210 mg
Cholesterol	0

Yield: 1 ½-cup serving

Food Exchange: ½ fruit

Festive Fruit Punch

1 46-ounce can pineapple juice
1 10-ounce package frozen raspberries, thawed
4 cups sugar-free lemonade
4 cups sugar-free lemon-lime drink
Lemon slices

Combine all ingredients. Garnish with lemon slices. Serve over ice.

Calories per serving	
Protein	41
Carbohydrate	0
Fat	10 g
Sodium	0
Potassium	0
Cholesterol	101 mg
	0

Yield: 20 ½-cup servings

Food Exchange: ½ fruit

Frozen Virgin Banana Daiquiri

2 ripe bananas, sliced
2 teaspoons rum extract
3 tablespoons lime juice
½ cup pineapple juice
5 to 6 packets sugar substitute
Ice cubes

Yield: 4 ½-cup servings

Food Exchange: 1 fruit

Combine all ingredients in a blender. Blend on high until thick and creamy.

Calories per serving	73
Protein	1 g
Carbohydrate	19 g
Fat	0
Sodium	0
Potassium	282 mg
Cholesterol	0

Peanut Butter Smoothee

2 cups pineapple juice
2 ripe bananas
2 tablespoons creamy peanut
  butter
2 tablespoons plain low-fat
  yogurt
Ice cubes

Yield: 6 ½-cup servings
Food Exchanges: 1½ fruits +
½ fat

Combine ingredients in a blender. Cover and blend until smooth.

Calories per serving	115
Protein	2 g
Carbohydrate	21 g
Fat	3 g
Sodium	36 mg
Potassium	306 mg
Cholesterol	0

4

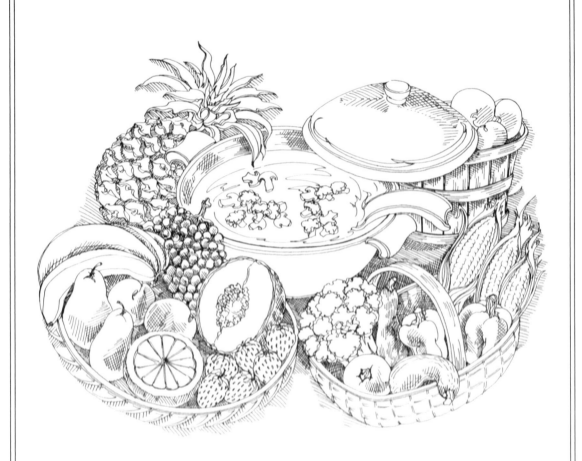

Soups, Salads, and Vegetables

Watercress Soup

2 green onions, minced
1 teaspoon vegetable oil
2 cups chopped watercress,
   stems removed
4 cups chicken stock
½ teaspoon ground coriander
15 green or black peppercorns
½ teaspoon salt
Grated Parmesan cheese

Yield: 4 1-cup servings

Food Exchange: 1 vegetable

Sauté onions in oil until clear and tender. Combine with remaining ingredients, except cheese, in a saucepan. Cook over medium heat for 30 minutes. Serve with Parmesan cheese sprinkled on top.

Calories per serving	25
Protein	1 g
Carbohydrate	1 g
Fat	1 g
Sodium	296 mg
Potassium	138 mg
Cholesterol	1 mg

Gazpacho

3 cups vegetable juice cocktail
   or tomato juice
2 tomatoes, peeled and
   chopped
1 cucumber, thinly sliced
½ cup finely chopped green
   pepper
¼ cup minced onion
2 teaspoons wine vinegar
1 clove garlic, minced
⅛ teaspoon ground white
   pepper
2 tablespoons minced fresh
   parsley

Yield: 8 ½-cup servings

Food Exchange: 1 vegetable

Combine all ingredients in a bowl. Chill at least 4 hours before serving.

Calories per serving	33
Protein	1 g
Carbohydrate	7 g
Fat	0
Sodium	257 mg
Potassium	316 mg
Cholesterol	0

Cucumber Soup

2 cups chicken stock
2 cups chopped cucumber
(seeds removed)
1 medium onion, chopped
¼ teaspoon salt
Dash cayenne pepper
2 tablespoons cornstarch
1 cup low-fat milk
Chopped parsley

Combine chicken stock, cucumbers, onion, salt, and pepper in a saucepan. Cover and simmer for 15 minutes, or until onion and cucumbers are tender. Purée in a blender. Dissolve cornstarch in milk and add to cucumber mixture. Heat over low heat just until thickened. Chill thoroughly. Serve cold. Garnish with parsley.

Calories per serving	45
Protein	2 g
Carbohydrate	8 g
Fat	1 g
Sodium	107 mg
Potassium	160 mg
Cholesterol	3 mg

Yield: 6 ½-cup servings

Food Exchanges: 2 vegetables

Purée of Broccoli Soup

1 pound fresh broccoli
3 cups chicken broth
5 green onions, chopped
Thin slices of lemon
Chopped fresh parsley

Chop broccoli. Simmer broccoli, chicken broth, and onions in a saucepan or slow cooker until tender. Purée in a food processor or blender. Serve with lemon slices and parsley.

Calories per serving	27
Protein	3 g
Carbohydrate	5 g
Fat	0
Sodium	11 mg
Potassium	304 mg
Cholesterol	0

Yield: 4 1-cup servings

Food Exchange: 1 vegetable

Bouillabaisse

1½ pounds fish (swordfish, scrod, or halibut)

1 pound shrimp or lobster tails

1 dozen clams or mussels

1 large onion, chopped

1 clove garlic, minced

1 16-ounce can tomatoes in juice

1 28-ounce can tomato purée

1 bay leaf

1 teaspoon dried thyme leaves

½ teaspoon dried rosemary

¼ teaspoon celery seeds

2 tablespoons chopped fresh parsley

Generous pinch saffron

2 cups water

Cut fish into 2-inch pieces. Peel shrimp or lobster tails. Wash clams. Combine all ingredients in a large kettle. Simmer for 15 to 20 minutes or until fish is tender and clam shells are open.

Calories per serving	184
Protein	27 g
Carbohydrate	9 g
Fat	4 g
Sodium	605 mg
Potassium	832 mg
Cholesterol	40 mg

Note: This recipe contains 400 milligrams or more of sodium per serving.

Yield: 8 1½-cup servings

Food Exchanges: 3 lean meats + 1 vegetable

Medley Vegetable Soup

4 cups chicken broth
1 turnip, peeled and diced
1 parsnip, peeled and diced
1 medium zucchini, sliced
6 carrots, peeled and sliced
2 stalks celery, chopped
1 cup fresh or frozen green
    beans, chopped
¼ cup chopped onion
1 cup fresh parsley sprigs
1 bay leaf
8 whole peppercorns
2 tablespoons fresh minced
    tarragon leaves or 1
    tablespoon dried tarragon
    leaves

Yield: 12 ½-cup servings

Food Exchange: 1 vegetable

Combine all ingredients in a saucepan or slow cooker. Cook until vegetables are tender.

Calories per serving	28
Protein	1 g
Carbohydrate	6 g
Fat	0
Sodium	30 mg
Potassium	227 mg
Cholesterol	0

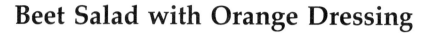

Beet Salad with Orange Dressing

6 large, fresh beets (about 2
  pounds)
¼ cup vegetable oil
¼ cup orange juice
2 tablespoons wine vinegar
Grated rind of 1 orange
1 packet sugar substitute
2 tablespoons chopped toasted
  walnuts

Yield: 6 ½-cup servings

Food Exchanges: 1 vegetable +
2 fats

Cook beets in water until tender, about 40 minutes. Rinse under cold water and peel off skin. Slice thin and cut into julienne strips. Combine oil, orange juice, vinegar, grated orange rind, and sugar substitute in a small bowl. Beat well. Pour dressing over beets. Toss. Refrigerate for 3 to 4 hours or overnight before serving. Sprinkle on walnuts.

Calories per serving	117
Protein	1 g
Carbohydrate	5 g
Fat	10 g
Sodium	101 mg
Potassium	103 mg
Cholesterol	0

Sweet-and-Sour Cucumbers

2 cucumbers, thinly sliced
2-inch piece fresh ginger,
  peeled and grated
1 packet sugar substitute
1 tablespoon sesame oil
1 tablespoon cider vinegar

Yield: 4 ½-cup servings

Food Exchange: ½ fat

Combine all ingredients in a bowl. Toss lightly. Chill thoroughly.

Calories per serving	36
Protein	0
Carbohydrate	1 g
Fat	3 g
Sodium	3 mg
Potassium	80 mg
Cholesterol	0

Watercress, Beet, and Orange Salad

4 medium beets (about 1
 pound)
2 bunches watercress
¼ cup fresh lemon juice
¼ cup vegetable oil
2 green onions, finely chopped
Pinch ground black pepper
1 orange

Cook beets in boiling water until tender. Meanwhile wash watercress and remove thick stems. Refrigerate until ready to serve. Combine lemon juice, oil, onions, and pepper in a bowl. Beat to blend flavors. When beets are tender, rinse under cold water and remove skins. Cut beets into julienne strips. Toss beets in lemon juice dressing. Peel orange and cut into small pieces. To serve, place watercress on serving dish. Top with beets, draining off excess dressing. Arrange orange pieces over beets. Toss together lightly to mix, if desired.

Yield: 6 ½-cup servings

Food Exchanges: 1 vegetable +
2 fats

Calories per serving	115
Protein	1 g
Carbohydrate	8 g
Fat	9 g
Sodium	144 mg
Potassium	182 mg
Cholesterol	0

Pea Salad

2 cups cooked or 1 10-ounce
 package frozen peas
1 cup chopped celery (1 stalk)
2 green onions, finely chopped
2 tablespoons mayonnaise
¼ teaspoon dill weed
½ teaspoon prepared mustard

Steam peas and celery until tender. Cool. Combine all ingredients in a bowl. Toss and refrigerate for 3 hours or overnight.

Yield: 4 ½-cup servings

Food Exchanges: 1 starch/bread
+ 1 fat

Calories per serving	108
Protein	5 g
Carbohydrate	10 g
Fat	6 g
Sodium	147 mg
Potassium	160 mg
Cholesterol	4 mg

Carrot and Grape Salad

4 large carrots, grated
1½ cups seedless green grapes
¼ cup toasted walnut halves
2 tablespoons vegetable oil
2 tablespoons wine vinegar
½ teaspoon prepared mustard

Yield: 8 ½-cup servings

Food Exchanges: 1 fruit + 1 fat

Combine all ingredients in a mixing bowl. Toss to mix well. Serve immediately.

Calories per serving	91
Protein	1 g
Carbohydrate	10 g
Fat	6 g
Sodium	22 mg
Potassium	197 mg
Cholesterol	0

Eggplant-Tomato Salad

1 medium eggplant, peeled
2 cups chopped tomatoes
1 cucumber, chopped
1 small green pepper, chopped
1 clove garlic, minced
4 green onions, chopped
¼ cup chopped fresh parsley
½ teaspoon dried oregano
  leaves
½ teaspoon dried basil leaves
¼ teaspoon ground black
  pepper
¼ cup olive oil
¼ cup wine vinegar

Yield: 8 ¾-cup servings

Food Exchanges: 1 vegetable + 1 fat

Cut eggplant into slices about ½-inch thick. Broil on a baking sheet about 4 minutes on each side until lightly browned. Cool. Cut into pieces. Combine all ingredients in a mixing bowl. Toss gently. Cover and refrigerate for at least 2 hours before serving.

Calories per serving	83
Protein	1 g
Carbohydrate	5 g
Fat	7 g
Sodium	4 mg
Potassium	230 mg
Cholesterol	0

Lobster Salad

1 pound lobster tail, cooked
1 tablespoon mayonnaise
½ teaspoon grated orange peel
⅓ cup thinly sliced celery
1 green onion, thinly sliced
2 oranges, peeled and
   sectioned

Yield: 2 ½-cup servings

Cut lobster meat into ½-inch pieces. Combine mayonnaise, orange peel, celery, and onion. Add lobster and orange sections. Toss lightly. Refrigerate for 30 minutes to blend flavors. Serve on lettuce.

Calories per serving	186
Protein	15 g
Carbohydrate	17 g
Fat	7 g
Sodium	224 mg
Potassium	185 mg
Cholesterol	91 mg

Kiwi and Hearts of Palm Salad

1 kiwi fruit
1 14-ounce can hearts of palm,
   drained
1 orange
Bibb lettuce or watercress
¼ cup toasted pine nuts
2 teaspoons walnut or
   vegetable oil
2 teaspoons red wine vinegar
Chopped fresh parsley

Yield: 4 ½-cup servings

Food Exchanges: 1 vegetable +
½ fruit

Peel and slice kiwi fruit. Cut hearts of palm into ½-inch pieces. Peel and slice orange. Arrange kiwi fruit slices, hearts of palm, and orange slices on lettuce. Add pine nuts. Drizzle on oil and vinegar. Sprinkle on parsley.

Calories per serving	84
Protein	2 g
Carbohydrate	10 g
Fat	2 g
Sodium	76 mg
Potassium	176 mg
Cholesterol	0

Apple-Pecan Salad

*2 cups bite-size pieces Granny
  Smith apples, cored*
*¼ cup broken pecan pieces,
  toasted*
¼ cup vanilla yogurt
1 tablespoon mayonnaise
1 packet sugar substitute
⅛ teaspoon ground cinnamon

Yield: 6 ½-cup servings

Food Exchanges: 1 fruit + 1 fat

Combine apples and pecans in bowl. Mix rest of the ingredients together and pour over apples. Toss gently to coat apples. Chill until ready to serve.

Calories per serving	111
Protein	1 g
Carbohydrate	16 g
Fat	6 g
Sodium	20 mg
Potassium	159 mg
Cholesterol	2 mg

Sunshine Delight

*1 0.3-ounce package sugar-free
  orange gelatin*
1 cup boiling water
*1 10¼-ounce can mandarin
  orange segments*
½ cup grated carrots
1 banana, peeled and sliced
½ cup cold water

Yield: 4 ½-cup servings

Food Exchange: 1 fruit

Dissolve gelatin in 1 cup boiling water as directed on package. Add remaining ingredients. Stir to blend. Pour into mold. Refrigerate until set.

Calories per serving	49
Protein	0
Carbohydrate	12 g
Fat	0
Sodium	8 mg
Potassium	234 mg
Cholesterol	0

Shrimp Slaw

2 tablespoons white wine
  vinegar
2 teaspoons white wine (Dijon)
  mustard
2 tablespoons vegetable oil
3 cups finely shredded cabbage
½ pound medium shrimp
¼ cup sliced almonds, toasted

In a large bowl, combine the vinegar and mustard. Add the oil in a stream, whisking until the dressing is thickened. Add the cabbage and toss to mix with the dressing. Chill. Cook shrimp in a covered saucepan in 1 cup boiling water for 2 minutes, or until pink. Drain the shrimp in a colander. Shell, devein, and cut shrimp in half lengthwise. Add the shrimp and almonds to the cabbage mixture. Toss well.

Yield: 4 1-cup servings

Food Exchanges: 2 lean meats + 1 fat

Calories per serving	153
Protein	13 g
Carbohydrate	4 g
Fat	10 g
Sodium	146 mg
Potassium	194 mg
Cholesterol	110 mg

Carrot-Raisin Salad

2 cups grated fresh carrots
½ cup raisins
¼ cup plain yogurt
¼ cup mayonnaise
½ packet sugar substitute

Combine all ingredients in a mixing bowl. Toss to blend thoroughly. Chill at least 1 hour before serving

Yield: 6 ⅓-cup servings

Food Exchanges: 1 vegetable + ½ fruit + 1½ fats

Calories per serving	123
Protein	2 g
Carbohydrate	14 g
Fat	8 g
Sodium	77 mg
Potassium	239 mg
Cholesterol	6 mg

Orange-Shrimp Salad

1 pound steamed shrimp
1 tablespoon chopped green onions
½ cup chopped celery
2 tablespoons olive oil
1 tablespoon wine vinegar
½ teaspoon dried rosemary, crumbled
⅛ teaspoon ground white pepper
4 navel oranges, peeled and sliced
Lettuce leaves

Peel shrimp. Combine onion, celery, oil, vinegar, rosemary, and pepper in a bowl. Mix well. Pour over shrimp. Chill. Place orange slices on lettuce leaves in serving dish. Add shrimp and dressing.

Calories per serving	198
Protein	18 g
Carbohydrate	17 g
Fat	8 g
Sodium	188 mg
Potassium	248 mg
Cholesterol	140 mg

Yield: 4 1-cup servings

Food Exchanges: 3 lean meats + 1 fruit

Two Bean–Orange Salad

1 10-ounce package frozen cut green beans
1 15-ounce can red kidney beans, drained
1 small onion, sliced into rings
2 navel oranges, peeled and sliced
¼ cup Italian dressing

Steam green beans until tender. Combine with remaining ingredients and refrigerate for 3 hours or overnight.

Calories per serving	164
Protein	5 g
Carbohydrate	21 g
Fat	7 g
Sodium	270 mg
Potassium	356 mg
Cholesterol	0

Yield: 4 ¾-cup servings

Food Exchanges: 1 starch/bread + 1 vegetable + 1 fat

Green Beans and Red Pepper Salad

1 pound fresh green beans or 1
  10-ounce package frozen
  green beans
1 sweet red or green pepper,
  cut into strips
1 small red onion, chopped
1 teaspoon mustard
1 tablespoon wine vinegar
2 tablespoons vegetable oil
¼ teaspoon ground cumin
2 tablespoons finely chopped
  fresh parsley

Steam green beans or defrost if frozen. Steam pepper strips. Combine green beans, peppers, and remaining ingredients in a covered bowl. Chill thoroughly.

Calories per serving	86
Protein	2 g
Carbohydrate	6 g
Fat	7 g
Sodium	23 mg
Potassium	158 mg
Cholesterol	0

Yield: 4 ½-cup servings

Food Exchanges: 1 vegetable +
1 fat

Apple–Sunflower Seed Salad

2 red apples, cored
1 green apple
¼ cup toasted unsalted
  sunflower seeds
¼ cup raisins
1 packet sugar substitute
2 teaspoons lemon juice

Grate apples. Combine all ingredients in a mixing bowl. Refrigerate until ready to serve.

Calories per serving	139
Protein	3 g
Carbohydrate	26 g
Fat	5 g
Sodium	5 mg
Potassium	274 mg
Cholesterol	0

Yield: 4 ¼-cup servings

Food Exchanges: 1½ fruits +
1 fat

Waldorf Salad

1 teaspoon mayonnaise
2 tablespoons plain yogurt
1 packet sugar substitute
3 red apples
½ cup chopped celery
¼ cup chopped walnuts,
    toasted

Yield: 4 ½-cup servings

Food Exchanges: 1 fruit + 1 fat

Combine mayonnaise, yogurt, and sugar substitute in a bowl. Add remaining ingredients. Toss lightly.

Calories per serving	125
Protein	2 g
Carbohydrate	18 g
Fat	6 g
Sodium	28 mg
Potassium	215 mg
Cholesterol	1 mg

Citrus Spaghetti Salad

4 ounces uncooked spaghetti
    noodles
2 cups broccoli pieces
½ cup sliced celery
2 green onions, finely chopped
2 oranges, peeled and sliced
2 tablespoons vegetable oil
2 tablespoons lemon juice
1 tablespoon mustard
1 packet sugar substitute
1 teaspoon dried tarragon
    leaves

Yield: 6 1-cup servings

Food Exchanges: 1 starch/bread
+ 1 vegetable + 1 fat

Break spaghetti noodles into thirds and cook as directed on package. Drain and cool. Steam broccoli. Add to cooked spaghetti noodles along with celery, onions, and oranges. Combine oil, lemon juice, mustard, sugar substitute, and tarragon in a bowl. Mix well. Pour over other ingredients. Toss gently but thoroughly. Chill.

Calories per serving	155
Protein	5 g
Carbohydrate	24 g
Fat	5 g
Sodium	37 mg
Potassium	268 mg
Cholesterol	0

Banana Salad

½ *piece grated fresh ginger root*
¼ *cup crème fraîche (see page 114)*
¼ *teaspoon ground nutmeg*
2 *tablespoons lemon juice*
¼ *cup plain yogurt*
2 *ripe bananas*
1 *apple, chopped*
2 *tablespoons toasted chopped pecans*

Combine ginger root, crème fraîche, nutmeg, lemon juice, and yogurt in a bowl. Peel and slice bananas into dressing. Add apple. Toss gently to coat banana and apple. Sprinkle pecan pieces on top. Serve immediately.

Calories per serving	153
Protein	2 g
Carbohydrate	20 g
Fat	8 g
Sodium	17 mg
Potassium	332 mg
Cholesterol	44 mg

Yield: 4 ¾-cup servings
Food Exchanges: 1 fruit + 2 fats

Pineapple-Grapefruit-Avocado Salad

1 *fresh pineapple, peeled*
2 *grapefruit, sectioned*
1 *cup sliced carrots, steamed*
8 to 10 *cherry tomatoes*
Fresh spinach leaves
1 *avocado, peeled and sliced*
¼ *cup vegetable oil*
2 *tablespoons vinegar*
3 *tablespoons pineapple juice*

Cut pineapple into quarters and remove core. Slice thin. Add grapefruit sections, carrots, and tomatoes. Just before serving, arrange fruit on spinach leaves. Top with avocado slices. Combine oil, vinegar, and pineapple juice in a bottle. Shake vigorously. Serve as a dressing with the salad.

Calories per serving	172
Protein	2 g
Carbohydrate	20 g
Fat	11 g
Sodium	14 mg
Potassium	426 mg
Cholesterol	0

Yield: 8 ½-cup servings

Food Exchanges: 1 fruit + 2 fats

Sesame-Fruit Salad

1 avocado, peeled and cubed
1 cup honeydew melon chunks
1 whole pineapple, peeled and cubed, or 1 cup juice-packed canned pineapple chunks
1 cup seedless grapes
1 tablespoon toasted sesame seeds

Yield: 8 ½-cup servings

Food Exchanges: 1 fruit + 1 fat

Combine all ingredients, except sesame seeds, in a mixing bowl. Toss to blend. Pour into a serving bowl. Sprinkle sesame seeds on fruit just before serving.

Calories per serving	111
Protein	1 g
Carbohydrate	19 g
Fat	5 g
Sodium	7 mg
Potassium	370 mg
Cholesterol	0

Pineapple and Cheese Delight

1 0.3-ounce package sugar-free lime gelatin
1 cup boiling water
1 8-ounce can crushed pineapple in juice
1 cup dry cottage cheese
¼ cup broken walnut pieces
½ cup cold water

Yield: 4 ½-cup servings

Food Exchanges: 1 lean meat + 1 fat

Dissolve gelatin in boiling water as directed on package. Add pineapple and juice, cottage cheese, walnut pieces, and cold water. Stir to mix. Pour into mold. Refrigerate until firm, at least 3 hours or overnight.

Calories per serving	115
Protein	8 g
Carbohydrate	11 g
Fat	5 g
Sodium	6 mg
Potassium	118 mg
Cholesterol	3 mg

Red, White, and Blue Salad

5 teaspoons (5 packages)
   unflavored gelatin
2½ cups low-calorie cranberry
   juice
4 packets sugar substitute
1 cup sliced fresh strawberries
1 cup part-skim ricotta cheese
1 cup fresh or frozen
   blueberries
1 cup (1 medium) banana slices

Sprinkle 2 teaspoons gelatin over 1 cup cranberry juice. Let stand for 5 minutes to soften gelatin. Cook over low heat until gelatin dissolves. Pour into a bowl and add 2 packets of sugar substitute. Chill until thickened like corn syrup. Stir in strawberries. Pour into a 6-cup mold. Refrigerate.

Make the second layer by dissolving 1 teaspoon gelatin in 1 cup cold water. Let stand for 5 minutes to soften gelatin. Cook over low heat until gelatin dissolves. Pour mixture into a food processor or blender. Add ricotta cheese and 1 packet of sugar substitute. Blend until smooth. Spoon ricotta mixture over strawberry layer. Refrigerate.

Make the third layer by sprinkling 2 teaspoons gelatin over 1½ cups cranberry juice. Let stand for 5 minutes to soften gelatin. Cook over low heat until gelatin dissolves. Chill until thickened like corn syrup. Stir in blueberries, banana, and remaining packet of sugar substitute. Spoon onto ricotta layer. Refrigerate until firm, at least 3 hours or overnight.

Calories per serving	64
Protein	3 g
Carbohydrate	8 g
Fat	3 g
Sodium	19 mg
Potassium	95 mg
Cholesterol	10 mg

Yield: 12 ½-cup servings

Food Exchanges: ½ fruit + ½ fat

Turkey-Chestnut Salad

*12 chestnuts, roasted and
    shelled*
3 cups chopped cooked turkey
¼ cup mayonnaise
1 tablespoon capers
1 teaspoon Dijon mustard
½ teaspoon anchovy paste
*½ teaspoon dried tarragon
    leaves*
1 apple, chopped

Yield: 6 1-cup servings

Food Exchanges: 3 medium-fat
meats

Cut chestnuts in half. Combine all ingredients in a bowl and toss to blend. Refrigerate for 1 hour. Serve on lettuce.

Calories per serving	220
Protein	21 g
Carbohydrate	5 g
Fat	13 g
Sodium	428 mg
Potassium	256 mg
Cholesterol	59 mg

Note: This recipe contains 400 milligrams or more of sodium per serving.

Brussels Sprouts and Hazelnuts

¼ cup hazelnuts, thinly sliced
1 tablespoon margarine
1 pound fresh Brussels sprouts

Yield: 4 ½-cup servings

Food Exchanges: 1 vegetable +
1½ fats

Sauté nuts in margarine. Steam Brussels sprouts. Combine nuts and sprouts in a serving bowl.

Calories per serving	103
Protein	3 g
Carbohydrate	6 g
Fat	8 g
Sodium	44 mg
Potassium	276 mg
Cholesterol	0

Green Beans and Mushrooms Almondine

6 large mushrooms
1 tablespoon margarine
½ pound fresh green beans
¼ cup slivered almonds,
  toasted

Slice mushrooms and sauté in margarine in a skillet until tender. Meanwhile steam green beans. Combine mushrooms, green beans, and almonds in skillet. Heat to blend flavors.

Calories per serving	91
Protein	3 g
Carbohydrate	5 g
Fat	7 g
Sodium	38 g
Potassium	191 mg
Cholesterol	0

Yield: 4 ½-cup servings

Food Exchanges: 1 vegetable + 1½ fats

Parsnips and Snow Peas

1 pound fresh parsnips
3 green onions, chopped
½ pound fresh snow peas
1 tablespoon sesame seeds,
  toasted

Peel parsnips and cut into lengthwise strips about 3 inches long. Sauté in a no-stick skillet with onions until parsnips are tender. Add snow peas. Sauté for another minute. Sprinkle sesame seeds on vegetables.

Calories per serving	50
Protein	2 g
Carbohydrate	11 g
Fat	1 g
Sodium	34 mg
Potassium	342 mg
Cholesterol	0

Yield: 4 ½-cup servings

Food Exchange: ½ starch/bread

Corn-Potato Hash

1 cup cooked fresh corn or 1
  16-ounce can whole kernel
  corn
1 teaspoon vegetable oil
½ cup chopped onion
½ cup chopped green pepper
2 medium potatoes, cooked
  and sliced
Dash ground white pepper
1 tablespoon chopped pimento
½ teaspoon salt (optional)

Yield: 4 ½-cup servings

Food Exchanges: 1 starch/bread
+ 2 vegetables

Food Exchanges: 1 lean meat +
1 starch/bread + 2 vegetables

Combine all ingredients in a skillet. Cook over medium heat about 10 minutes, or until mixture is hot.

Calories per serving	119
Protein	4 g
Carbohydrate	25 g
Fat	2 g
Sodium	105 mg
Potassium	367 mg
Cholesterol	0

Vegetarian Entrée: Sprinkle 1 cup grated low-fat mozzarella cheese over top before serving.

Calories per serving	159
Protein	8 g
Carbohydrate	25 g
Fat	4 g
Sodium	171 mg
Potassium	380 mg
Cholesterol	8 mg

Spiced Cauliflower

2 tablespoons vegetable oil
2 teaspoons mustard seeds
2-inch piece fresh ginger root
½ teaspoon turmeric powder
2 teaspoons cumin seeds
1 head cauliflower, separated
  into florets
¼ teaspoon paprika
¼ teaspoon ground black
  pepper
½ teaspoon salt
2 to 4 tablespoons coconut
  milk
2 red dried chilies, seeded and
  minced (optional)

Combine oil and mustard seeds in a skillet. Fry until seeds pop. Peel and mince gingerroot. Add to mustard seeds with turmeric powder. Sauté over medium flame for 2 minutes. Stir in remaining ingredients, except chilies. Cover and cook over low heat about 10 minutes or until cauliflower is tender. Sprinkle on chilies just before serving.

Calories per serving	59
Protein	2 g
Carbohydrate	4 g
Fat	5 g
Sodium	172 mg
Potassium	197 mg
Cholesterol	0

Yield: 6 ½-cup servings

Food Exchanges: 1 vegetable + 1 fat

Baby Carrots à la Mint

1 pound small carrots (about
  20)
1 green onion, chopped
1 tablespoon margarine
1 tablespoon chopped fresh
  mint leaves or 1½ teaspoons
  dried mint leaves

Peel carrots. Steam carrots with green onion until tender. Add margarine and mint leaves.

Calories per serving	36
Protein	1 g
Carbohydrate	5 g
Fat	2 g
Sodium	42 mg
Potassium	187 mg
Cholesterol	0

Yield: 8 ½-cup servings

Food Exchange: 1 vegetable

Red Potatoes in Parchment

4 medium red potatoes
½ cup sliced fresh mushrooms
  (about 8)
2 cloves garlic, minced
4 sprigs parsley
½ teaspoon dried sage leaves
½ teaspoon dried oregano
  leaves
2 teaspoons olive oil

Yield: 4 servings

Food Exchanges: 2 starches/
breads

Slice potatoes onto four pieces of parchment paper measuring 16-by-12 inches each. Divide remaining ingredients among each potato mixture. Seal paper by tightly folding edges. Place on a baking sheet and bake in a 400-degree oven for 18 to 20 minutes, or over medium coals for 20 to 25 minutes.

Calories per serving	148
Protein	4 g
Carbohydrate	28 g
Fat	2 g
Sodium	6 mg
Potassium	580 mg
Cholesterol	0

Glazed Sweet Potatoes

2½ pounds fresh sweet
  potatoes, peeled
2 tablespoons margarine
1 tablespoon brown sugar
2 tablespoons chopped pecans

Yield: 8 servings

Food Exchanges: 1 starch/bread
+ 1 fat

Cut sweet potatoes into quarters and cook in boiling water just until tender. Drain. Place potato pieces in a baking dish and top with margarine, brown sugar, and pecans. Bake in a 350-degree oven for 15 to 18 minutes, or until pecans are toasted.

Calories per serving	98
Protein	1 g
Carbohydrate	14 g
Fat	4 g
Sodium	37 mg
Potassium	139 mg
Cholesterol	0

Spaghetti Squash Confetti

1 3-pound spaghetti squash
1 tablespoon olive oil
1 tablespoon wine vinegar
1 tablespoon chopped pimento
½ cup chopped green pepper
¼ cup chopped onion
1 small clove garlic, minced
¼ teaspoon ground cumin
¼ cup minced fresh parsley

Yield: 4 ½-cup servings

Food Exchanges: 1 starch/bread
+ 1 fat

Cook squash in a microwave oven, a conventional oven, or by steaming in a saucepan. Split and remove seeds. Pull out flesh with a fork. Reserve shell. Toss to separate strands. Add remaining ingredients and stuff into shell. Bake in a 350-degree oven for 10 to 15 minutes or until hot. Serve warm or cold.

Calories per serving	103
Protein	3 g
Carbohydrate	18 g
Fat	4 g
Sodium	5 mg
Potassium	524 mg
Cholesterol	0

Pickled Beets

1 cup sliced cooked beets
1 small onion, sliced
¼ cup cider vinegar
1 packet sugar substitute

Yield: 4 ¼-cup servings

Food Exchange: 1 vegetable

Combine all ingredients in a mixing bowl. Refrigerate at least 1 hour before serving.

Calories per serving	24
Protein	1 g
Carbohydrate	5 g
Fat	0
Sodium	102 mg
Potassium	103 mg
Cholesterol	0

Zucchini Casserole

1 large zucchini (1 pound),
*   sliced*
1 medium onion, chopped
½ teaspoon dried oregano
*   leaves*
½ teaspoon dried basil leaves
2 tablespoons vegetable oil
2 cloves garlic, minced
1 egg
1 tablespoon fresh minced
*   parsley*
¼ cup grated Parmesan or
*   Romano cheese*
⅛ teaspoon ground white
*   pepper*

Sauté zucchini, onion, garlic, oregano, and basil in oil until zucchini is tender. Spoon into a lightly oiled casserole dish. Combine remaining ingredients. Pour over zucchini. Bake in a 350-degree oven 15 to 20 minutes, or until browned. Let stand for 5 minutes before serving.

Calories per serving	129
Protein	5 g
Carbohydrate	5 g
Fat	10 g
Sodium	114 mg
Potassium	202 mg
Cholesterol	72 mg

Yield: 4 ½-cup servings

Food Exchanges: 1 vegetable +
2 fats

5

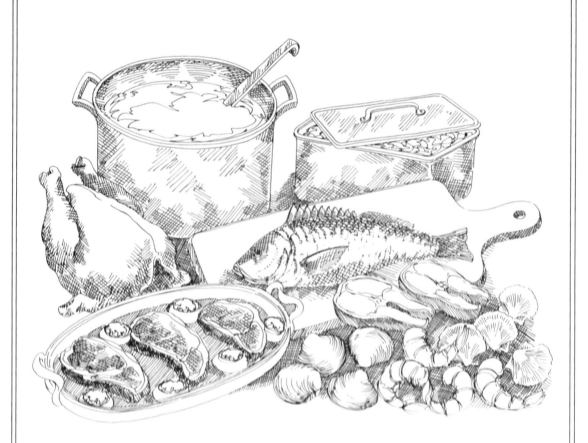

Fish, Poultry, and Meats

Baked Fish with Tomato-Pepper Sauce

1 tablespoon vegetable oil
2 medium onions, chopped
2 red bell peppers, chopped
1 small hot pepper, seeds
  discarded
3 cloves garlic, chopped
2 pounds ripe tomatoes, peeled
  and seeded, or 2 28-ounce
  cans tomatoes, drained and
  chopped
1½ to 2 pounds fillets of
  halibut, cod, sole, or
  haddock

Yield: 6 servings of 1 fillet

Food Exchanges: 3 lean meats +
1 vegetable

Heat oil in a skillet. Add onions, peppers, and garlic. Cook until peppers are soft. Add tomatoes and cook until sauce is thick. Spread sauce in the bottom of a large shallow baking pan. Arrange fish fillets on top. Spoon a layer of sauce on top of each fillet. Bake in a 425-degree oven for 12 to 15 minutes, or until fish is tender and flakes when tested with a fork.

Calories per serving	190
Protein	22 g
Carbohydrate	8 g
Fat	8 g
Sodium	118 mg
Potassium	745 mg
Cholesterol	54 mg

Gefilte Fish Loaf

2 pounds whitefish or turbot
  fillets
2 medium onions, finely
  chopped
2 carrots, grated
¼ cup matzo meal
1 teaspoon vegetable oil
¼ teaspoon salt
½ teaspoon ground nutmeg
2 whole eggs

Yield: 10 1-inch slice servings

Food Exchanges: 3 lean meats
+1 vegetable

Process fish in a food processor or blender until a paste forms. Combine fish with remaining ingredients. Pack mixture into a lightly oiled or no-stick 9-by-5-by-3-inch loaf pan. Bake in a 350-degree oven for 1 hour. Cool in pan. Turn out and refrigerate until ready to serve.

Calories per serving	179
Protein	22 g
Carbohydrate	5 g
Fat	7 g
Sodium	232 mg
Potassium	489 mg
Cholesterol	98 mg

Creamed Scallops and Lobster

2 tablespoons margarine
3 tablespoons unbleached flour
½ teaspoon salt
¼ teaspoon white pepper
½ teaspoon ground mustard
¼ teaspoon paprika
1 ½ cups skim milk
1 cup chopped celery
½ cup chopped green pepper
1 pound fresh or frozen bay
  scallops
½ pound cooked lobster
  chunks or shrimp
¼ grated Cheddar cheese

Melt margarine in a skillet. Add flour, salt, pepper, mustard, and paprika. Stir to make a paste. Add milk and mix well. Blend in celery and green pepper. When mixture thickens, add scallops. Cook about 3 minutes. Stir in lobster. Heat for 1 minute. Pour into a serving dish. Sprinkle cheese on top. Serve over toast points, rice, or noodles.*

Calories per serving	240
Protein	25 g
Carbohydrate	7 g
Fat	11 g
Sodium	589 mg
Potassium	529 mg
Cholesterol	85 mg

Yield: 6 ½-cup servings

Food Exchanges: 3 lean meats + 1 vegetable + ½ fat

Note: This recipe contains 400 milligrams or more of sodium per serving.

*Toast points, rice, or noodles are not included in the nutrient analysis for this recipe. One-third cup of cooked rice or ½ cup of cooked noodles equals 1 starch/bread exchange.

Crab Imperial

¼ *cup mayonnaise*
1 egg
2 tablespoons chopped green
  onion
2 tablespoons chopped
  pimento
2 teaspoons lemon juice
½ *teaspoon prepared mustard*
⅛ *teaspoon ground cayenne*
  pepper
1 pound cooked crabmeat
Paprika

Yield: 4 ½-cup servings

Food Exchanges: 2 lean meats +
1½ fats

Combine all ingredients, except paprika, in a mixing bowl. Stir gently to blend. Spoon into lightly oiled scallop dishes or individual casseroles. Sprinkle paprika on top. Bake in a 350-degree oven for 15 to 18 minutes.

Calories per serving	192
Protein	15 g
Carbohydrate	1 g
Fat	14 g
Sodium	104 mg
Potassium	488 mg
Cholesterol	102 mg

Wild Rice

¼ *cup chopped onion or*
  scallions
1 tablespoon margarine
⅛ *teaspoon ground sage*
⅛ *teaspoon dried thyme leaves*
⅛ *teaspoon dried marjoram*
  leaves
1 cup cooked wild rice

Yield: 2 ½-cup servings

Food Exchanges: 2 starches/
breads

Sauté onion in margarine until tender. Add sage, thyme, marjoram, and rice. Simmer over low heat 10 to 15 minutes for flavors to blend. Serve with Cornish hen, chicken, or venison.

Calories per serving	175
Protein	3 g
Carbohydrate	27 g
Fat	6 g
Sodium	344 mg
Potassium	104 mg
Cholesterol	0

Linguine with Clam Sauce

1 large clove garlic, minced
2 teaspoons olive oil
1 cup sliced mushrooms
1 10-ounce can minced clams
¼ cup white wine
¼ cup chopped fresh parsley
¼ teaspoon dried basil leaves
¼ teaspoon dried oregano
*   leaves*
4 ounces uncooked linguine
*   noodles*

Yield: 4 1½-cup servings

Food Exchanges: 2 lean meats +
2 starches/breads

Sauté garlic in oil. Add mushrooms and cook until tender. Stir in clams with juice, wine, parsley, basil, and oregano. Cook for 5 minutes or until liquids are reduced. Meanwhile, cook linguine and drain. Toss sauce with noodles just before serving.

Calories per serving	246
Protein	14 g
Carbohydrate	37 g
Fat	3 g
Sodium	160 mg
Potassium	391 mg
Cholesterol	89 mg

Shrimp Fried Rice

2 eggs
1 tablespoon vegetable oil
½ pound small, cooked, and
*   shelled shrimp*
2 cups cooked rice
½ cup frozen green peas

Yield: 4 servings of 8 shrimp

Food Exchanges: 1 starch/bread
+ 3 lean meats + 1 fat

Beat eggs. Heat oil in a wok or an electric skillet. Add shrimp, rice, and peas. Toss gently to heat over high temperature. Add eggs. Stir gently to cook eggs. Serve immediately.

Calories per serving	273
Protein	17 g
Carbohydrate	28 g
Fat	10 g
Sodium	545 mg
Potassium	232 mg
Cholesterol	137 mg

Note: This recipe contains 400 milligrams or more of sodium per serving.

Shrimp and Rice Cajun Style

1 pound fresh or frozen shrimp
1 tablespoon vegetable oil
1 clove garlic, minced
⅛ teaspoon ground cayenne
  pepper
¼ teaspoon ground black
  pepper
1 teaspoon dried thyme leaves
½ teaspoon dried basil leaves
½ teaspoon dried oregano
  leaves
½ cup tomato juice
1 large tomato, chopped
1 green pepper, chopped
1 ⅓ cups cooked rice

Peel and devein shrimp. Combine oil, garlic, cayenne and black peppers, thyme, basil, and oregano in a skillet over high heat. Add tomato juice, tomato, green pepper, and shrimp. Cover and cook for 5 minutes, or until shrimp are pink. Serve over rice.

Calories per serving	216
Protein	20 g
Carbohydrate	25 g
Fat	4 g
Sodium	560 mg
Potassium	418 mg
Cholesterol	165 mg

Yield: 4 1½-cup servings

Food Exchanges: 3 lean meats + 1 starch/bread + 2 vegetables

Note: This recipe contains 400 milligrams or more of sodium per serving.

Shrimp Almondine

1 pound fresh or frozen
* medium shrimp*
1 tablespoon margarine
¼ cup sliced almonds
3 green onions, finely chopped
Fresh chopped parsley

Shell and devein shrimp. Melt margarine in a skillet. Add almonds and sauté until browned. Remove almonds. Add shrimp and green onions. Cook just until shrimp are pink and tender, stirring constantly. Serve shrimp on noodles or rice.* Sprinkle almonds and parsley on top.

Calories per serving	113
Protein	17 g
Carbohydrate	0 g
Fat	5 g
Sodium	187 mg
Potassium	162 mg
Cholesterol	87 mg

Yield: 4 ½-cup servings

Food Exchange: 2 lean meats

*Rice or noodles are not included in the nutrient analysis for this recipe. One-third cup of cooked rice or ½ cup of cooked noodles equals 1 starch/bread exchange.

Shrimp Scampi

½ *pound large shrimp*
1 *tablespoon vegetable oil*
1 *small clove garlic, minced*
3 *green onions, finely chopped*
½ *lemon*
¼ *cup apple juice*
1 *tablespoon fresh minced*
  parsley

Shell and devein shrimp. Sauté oil, garlic, shrimp, and onions over low heat. Squeeze lemon over shrimp. Add apple juice. Cover and cook over low heat for 4 to 5 minutes, or until shrimp are pink. Sprinkle parsley on top just before serving with rice or linguine.*

Calories per serving	206
Protein	22 g
Carbohydrate	3 g
Fat	8 g
Sodium	211 mg
Potassium	364 mg
Cholesterol	120 mg

Yield: 2 ½-cup servings

Food Exchanges: 3 lean meats

* Rice or linguine is not included in the nutrient analysis for this recipe. One-third cup of cooked rice or ½ cup of cooked linguine equals 1 starch/bread exchange.

Spicy Baked Catfish

2 *pounds fresh or frozen whole*
  dressed catfish
1 *tablespoon vegetable oil*
1 *clove garlic, minced*
1 *tablespoon fennel seeds*
½ *teaspoon ground black*
  pepper
½ *teaspoon dried thyme leaves*
½ *teaspoon dried basil leaves*

Thaw catfish, if frozen. Combine oil and remaining ingredients in a skillet. Brown over medium heat. Add catfish. Brown on both sides. Put fish into a baking dish and bake in a 375-degree oven for 20 minutes, or until fish flakes when tested with a fork.

Calories per serving	125
Protein	21 g
Carbohydrate	2 g
Fat	5 g
Sodium	61 mg
Potassium	401 mg
Cholesterol	75 mg

Yield: 4 servings of ½ catfish

Food Exchanges: 3 lean meats

Scallops Ratatouille

2 cloves garlic, minced
1 large onion, thinly sliced
1 tablespoon olive oil
2 pounds medium zucchini,
  thinly sliced
1 pound eggplant, cubed
1 green pepper, cut into pieces
2 8-ounce cans tomatoes or 1
  pound fresh tomatoes, peeled
1 teaspoon dried basil leaves
½ teaspoon dried marjoram
  leaves
2 bay leaves
1 teaspoon freshly grated
  Parmesan cheese
1 teaspoon salt (optional)
1 pound fresh or frozen sea or
  bay scallops

Yield: 4 ¾-cup servings

Food Exchanges: 3 lean meats +
3 vegetables

Sauté garlic and onion in oil until tender. Add remaining ingredients, except scallops and Parmesan cheese. Break up tomatoes. Cook over medium heat for 20 minutes or until vegetables are tender. Add scallops and cook over medium heat just until tender, about 5 minutes. Sprinkle cheese on top just before serving. Serve with rice, if desired.*

Calories per serving	196
Protein	24 g
Carbohydrate	14 g
Fat	5 g
Sodium	403 mg
Potassium	1001 mg
Cholesterol	48 mg

Note: This recipe contains 400 milligrams or more of sodium per serving.

* Rice is not included in the nutrient analysis for this recipe. One-third cup of cooked rice equals 1 starch/bread exchange.

Scallops Pasta Salad

1 pound bay scallops
1 cup clam juice
1 8-ounce package seashell
   macaroni
½ cup plain low-fat yogurt
⅓ cup mayonnaise
1 tablespoon lemon juice
1 cup chopped celery
8 green onions, chopped
1 10-ounce package frozen
   peas, defrosted
1 cup low-fat cheese, cubed
1 cup chopped green pepper
2 tablespoons chopped
   pimento

Poach scallops in clam juice or fish broth just until tender, about 3 minutes. Cook macaroni according to package directions. Chill scallops and macaroni overnight. Add remaining ingredients. Toss gently to mix.

Calories per serving	319
Protein	21 g
Carbohydrate	38 g
Fat	9 g
Sodium	270 mg
Potassium	681 mg
Cholesterol	78 mg

Yield: 8 1½-cup servings

Food Exchanges: 2 lean meats + 2 starches/breads + 1 vegetable

Sweet-and-Sour Salmon

Salmon

¾ cup lemon juice

½ cup vinegar

3 onions, thinly sliced

½ cup raisins

¼ cup brown sugar

1 teaspoon ground ginger

2 tablespoons mixed whole
   pickling spices

3 cups water

3 pounds salmon fillets,
   skinned

Dill Sauce

¼ cup mayonnaise

2 tablespoons mustard

1 packet sugar substitute

1 teaspoon vinegar

3 tablespoons chopped fresh
   dill or 1 tablespoon dried dill
   weed

Yield: 10 3-strip servings

Food Exchanges: 3 medium-fat
meats

To prepare Salmon, combine lemon juice, vinegar, onions, raisins, brown sugar, ginger, and pickling spices and water in a large enamel or stainless steel saucepan. Bring to a boil. Cut salmon into 2-inch strips. Add salmon to pickling mixture and reduce heat to low. Cook for 30 minutes. Turn off heat; cool and refrigerate until ready to serve.

To prepare dill sauce, combine all ingredients in a mixing bowl. Blend well using a wire whisk.

Remove salmon strips from pickling mixture. Serve with 1 teaspoon dill sauce per serving.

Calories per serving	206
Protein	24 g
Carbohydrate	0
Fat	11 g
Sodium	173 mg
Potassium	406 mg
Cholesterol	45 mg

Salmon with Orange Sauce

1 pound salmon fillets
1 orange
1 tablespoon vegetable oil
Fresh chopped parsley

Rinse salmon fillets. Grate orange for 2 teaspoons rind. Squeeze orange for juice. Sauté fillets in a skillet with oil. Add orange rind and juice. Simmer until fish flakes when tested with a fork. Serve with parsley sprinkled on top.

Yield: 4 servings of 1 salmon fillet

Food Exchanges: 3 lean meats

Calories per serving	185
Protein	21 g
Carbohydrate	4 g
Fat	9 g
Sodium	109 mg
Potassium	488 mg
Cholesterol	54 mg

Rainbow Trout with Saffron Rice Stuffing

2 fresh or frozen rainbow trout
(about 1½ pounds each),
dressed
1 tablespoon vegetable oil
½ cup thinly sliced celery
3 green onions, finely chopped
2 inches fresh ginger, peeled
and minced
½ cup uncooked rice
¼ teaspoon saffron

Place each trout on a large piece of parchment paper in a baking pan. Sauté oil, celery, onions, and ginger until celery is tender. Cook rice according to package directions, adding saffron to water. Boil until tender. Drain off any water. Combine rice and celery mixture. Toss to blend. Spoon stuffing into each trout. Tightly seal parchment paper edges. Bake in a 400-degree oven for 18 to 20 minutes. Serve by cutting off top of parchment pouch.

Yield: 6 servings of ⅓ trout

Food Exchanges: ½ starch/bread + 3 lean meats

Calories per serving	228
Protein	26 g
Carbohydrate	9 g
Fat	9 g
Sodium	361 mg
Potassium	544 mg
Cholesterol	55 mg

Baked Trout with Clams

3½ to 4 pounds fresh trout,
  with heads and tails
1 cup fresh or canned
  tomatoes, skinned
¼ cup fresh chopped parsley
¼ cup finely chopped green
  onions
2 cloves garlic, finely chopped
1 teaspoon dried oregano
¼ teaspoon dried basil
¼ teaspoon salt
¼ teaspoon white pepper
1 bay leaf
½ cup dry white wine
12 cherrystone clams

Yield: 4 servings

Food Exchanges: 3 lean meats

Clean trout and score across top by making ¼-inch slashes. Place in a lightly oiled pan. Be sure to oil heads and tails to prevent drying and curling. Combine tomatoes, parsley, onion, garlic, oregano, basil, salt, pepper, and bay leaf in a mixing bowl. Spread mixture over fish. Add wine around sides of fish. Bake in a 400-degree oven for 15 minutes. Scrub clams. Place around fish in the baking dish and continue baking for 15 minutes, or until clams open.

Calories per serving	225
Protein	22 g
Carbohydrate	10 g
Fat	4 g
Sodium	108 mg
Potassium	516 mg
Cholesterol	69 mg

Paella

1 dozen small hard-shell clams

½ cup water

12 chicken legs

2 tablespoons olive or
  vegetable oil

1 onion, chopped

1 green pepper, chopped

1 clove garlic, minced

1 35-ounce can tomatoes,
  broken up

1 cup uncooked brown rice

1 teaspoon saffron

2 bay leaves

1 teaspoon dried basil leaves

½ teaspoon dried thyme leaves

½ teaspoon dried oregano
  leaves

1 10-ounce box frozen peas

12 large raw shrimp, shelled

Fresh chopped parsley or
  cilantro

Place clams and water in a saucepan. Bring to a boil. Cover and reduce heat to low. Cook until shells open, about 5 minutes. Remove from heat and cool. Reserve liquid. Remove skin from chicken legs. Heat oil in a skillet and add chicken. Brown chicken on all sides. Remove from the pan. Add onion, pepper, and garlic to oil. Sauté until onion is soft. Add tomatoes, rice, saffron, bay leaves, basil, thyme, and oregano. Stir to blend flavors. Spoon rice mixture into a large casserole. Arrange chicken over rice. Measure clam liquid. Add enough water to make 1 cup. Pour over rice. Sprinkle peas on top. Cover casserole and bake in a 350-degree oven for 55 to 60 minutes.

Remove from the oven and stir mixture. Place shrimp on top. Cover and bake for 10 more minutes, or until shrimp are pink. Uncover and place clams on top of rice. Return to the oven for 5 more minutes until clams are heated. Serve with fresh chopped parsley sprinkled on top.

Yield: 6 servings

Food Exchanges: 4 lean meats +
1 starch/bread + 2 vegetables

Calories per serving	318
Protein	27 g
Carbohydrate	27 g
Fat	12 g
Sodium	347 mg
Potassium	719 mg
Cholesterol	56 mg

Sesame-Baked Red Snapper

1 egg white, beaten
2 teaspoons Worcestershire
  sauce
⅛ Tabasco
1 teaspoon minced garlic or
  onion
1 pound fresh or frozen red
  snapper fillets
2 tablespoons sesame seeds
¼ cup cornflakes crumbs

Combine egg white, Worcestshire sauce, Tabasco, and garlic in a shallow dish. Stir to blend. Pour over fillets. Marinate at least 30 minutes or overnight in the refrigerator. Combine sesame seeds and corn-flakes crumbs. Roll fillets in mixture. Place fillets in an oiled shallow baking pan. Bake in a 350-degree oven for 15 to 20 minutes, or until browned and fish flakes when tested with a fork.

Yield: 3 servings of 1 fillet

Food Exchanges: 4 lean meats +
½ starch/bread

Calories per serving	247
Protein	30 g
Carbohydrate	9 g
Fat	9 g
Sodium	290 mg
Potassium	480 mg
Cholesterol	73 mg

Fresh Tuna Steaks

1 pound fresh tuna steaks
¼ cup Italian dressing
1 teaspoon margarine
2 tablespoons chopped green
  onions
1 tablespoon finely chopped
  parsley

Marinate tuna steaks in dressing for at least 30 minutes. Sauté margarine, green onions, and pars-ley in a skillet. Add tuna steaks. Brown on both sides. Cover with a lid and sauté for 5 to 10 minutes, depending on thickness of steak. Serve immedi-ately.

Yield: 4 servings of 1 tuna steak

Food Exchanges: 3 lean meats

Calories per serving	201
Protein	24 g
Carbohydrate	2 g
Fat	10 g
Sodium	164 mg
Potassium	10 mg
Cholesterol	71 mg

Vegetable Confetti Orange Roughy

*1 small red pepper, thinly
sliced*
1 small zucchini, shredded
1 small onion, thinly sliced
*1 8-ounce can water chestnuts,
chopped*
*2 tablespoons chopped fresh
parsley or 2 teaspoons dried
parsley flakes*
*1 teaspoon freshly grated
ginger root*
1 tablespoon margarine
*1 pound orange roughy or sole
fillets*

Yield: 4 servings of 1 fillet with
¼ cup topping

Food Exchanges: 3 lean meats +
1 vegetable

Sauté all ingredients, except fish fillets, in a skillet until onion is tender. Arrange fillets in a baking dish. Spread vegetables on top. Cover and bake in a 350-degree oven for 10 to 15 minutes, or until fish flakes when tested with a fork.

Calories per serving	161
Protein	22 g
Carbohydrate	8 g
Fat	4 g
Sodium	261 mg
Potassium	543 mg
Cholesterol	74 mg

Fillet of Sole Florentine

1 pound fillet of sole or
  flounder
2 cups water
2 bay leaves
1 onion, sliced
1 lemon, sliced
12 peppercorns
1 pound fresh spinach or 1
  10-ounce package frozen
  chopped spinach
1 egg yolk
2 tablespoons skim milk
2 tablespoons grated Parmesan
  cheese

Yield: 4 servings of 1 fillet

Food Exchanges: 4 lean meats +
1 vegetable

Place fillets in a skillet. Combine water, bay leaves, onion, lemon, and peppercorns in a saucepan. Cook over medium heat for 15 minutes to extract flavorings. Pour liquid over fish. Cover and simmer for 12 to 15 minutes, or until fish flakes when tested with a fork. Cook spinach in a steamer until tender. Drain well. Place spinach in the bottom of a casserole. Put fish fillets on top. Pour on sauce made from beating together egg yolk, milk, and cheese. Place under broiler until sauce is lightly browned.

Calories per serving	227
Protein	30 g
Carbohydrate	5 g
Fat	10 g
Sodium	295 mg
Potassium	799 mg
Cholesterol	125 mg

Greek Swordfish Steaks

*1 pound fresh or frozen
  swordfish steaks*
1 tablespoon olive oil
½ teaspoon dried oregano
¼ cup chopped green onions
*2 tablespoons chopped fresh
  parsley*
2 cloves garlic, minced
1 small onion, thinly sliced
1 lemon, thinly sliced
1 tomato, thinly sliced

Yield: 3 servings of 1 swordfish
steak

Food Exchanges: 4 lean meats +
1 vegetable

Place swordfish in an oiled shallow baking dish. Pour oil over fish. Sprinkle on oregano. Top with green onions, parsley, and garlic. Cover and bake for 10 minutes in a 350-degree oven. Remove from the oven and add onion, lemon, and tomato slices. Cover and bake for another 10 minutes, or until fish flakes when tested with a fork.

Calories per serving	207
Protein	29 g
Carbohydrate	6 g
Fat	7 g
Sodium	46 mg
Potassium	510 mg
Cholesterol	72 mg

Minted Lamb Roast with Apples

2 pounds lamb roast
1 tablespoon dried mint leaves
Juice of 1 lemon
2 apples, cut into wedges

Yield: 6 servings of 3 1-ounce
slices

Food Exchanges: 3 lean meats +
½ fruit

Place lamb roast in a baking pan. Sprinkle on mint leaves. Pour lemon juice over roast. Add apples along side. Roast in a 325-degree oven for 1½ hours or until tender.

Calories per serving	185
Protein	25 g
Carbohydrate	7 g
Fat	6 g
Sodium	60 mg
Potassium	326 mg
Cholesterol	90 mg

Lamb and Bean Stew

1 pound lamb cubes
½ cup chopped onion
½ cup water
1 clove garlic, minced
1 bay leaf
½ teaspoon dried oregano
   leaves
¼ teaspoon dried basil leaves
¼ teaspoon ground black
   pepper
2 cups canned great northern
   beans
1 tablespoon dried parsley
   flakes
1 tablespoon lemon juice
Lemon slices

Brown lamb and onion in a no-stick skillet. Add water, garlic, bay leaf, oregano, basil, and pepper. Cover and simmer for 1 hour. Add beans and parsley. Cover and cook 30 minutes longer or until lamb is tender. Stir in lemon juice. Pour into a serving dish. Garnish with slices of lemon.

Calories per serving	190
Protein	22 g
Carbohydrate	16 g
Fat	4 g
Sodium	46 mg
Potassium	483 mg
Cholesterol	60 mg

Yield: 6 1-cup servings

Food Exchanges: 2 lean meats +
1 starch/bread

Lamb Curry

1 pound cooked lamb cubes
1 small onion, chopped
1 clove garlic, minced
1 apple, chopped
1 to 1½ tablespoons curry
   powder
½ cup apple juice
Rice
Orange slices
Raisins
Chopped peanuts or cashews

Yield: 4 ½-cup servings

Food Exchanges: 3 lean meats +
1 vegetable

Cook lamb, onion, garlic, apple, and curry powder in apple juice until onion is soft. Serve over rice. Arrange orange slices, raisins, and peanuts on top or pass around in small serving bowls.*

Calories per serving	187
Protein	25 g
Carbohydrate	7 g
Fat	6 g
Sodium	63 mg
Potassium	349 mg
Cholesterol	90 mg

* Rice and accompaniments are not included in the nutrient analysis for this recipe. One-third cup of cooked rice equals 1 starch/bread exchange. Use small amounts of accompaniments as allowed in your individual meal plan.

Pork Roast with Quince

3 pounds pork roast
1 teaspoon dried thyme leaves
1 cup apple juice
4 potatoes, quartered
4 carrots, cut into chunks
2 stalks celery, cut into chunks
1 onion, sliced thick
1 quince or apple, cut into
   slices

Yield: 6 servings of 4 1-ounce slices with ⅔ cup vegetables

Food Exchanges: 4 lean meats +
1 starch/bread + 1 fruit

Sprinkle pork roast with thyme. Place in a baking pan. Add remaining ingredients around roast. Cover with a lid or foil. Bake in a 325-degree oven for 2 hours, or until roast is done.

Calories per serving	345
Protein	28 g
Carbohydrate	33 g
Fat	12 g
Sodium	98 mg
Potassium	954 mg
Cholesterol	78 mg

Pork Tenderloin Dijon

1 pound pork tenderloin
1 teaspoon vegetable oil
1 small onion, finely chopped
½ sweet red pepper, thinly
  sliced
1 tablespoon dijon mustard
½ cup apple juice
1 tablespoon capers
Chopped fresh thyme leaves*

Yield: 4 servings

Food Exchanges: 3 medium-fat meats + 1 vegetable

Cut tenderloin into ½ inch thick slices. Brown in oil over medium heat. Add onion, pepper, mustard, and apple juice. Cover and cook for 15 to 20 minutes, or until pork is tender. Add capers. Sprinkle with thyme just before serving.

Calories per serving	241
Protein	25 g
Carbohydrate	6 g
Fat	12 g
Sodium	111 mg
Potassium	408 mg
Cholesterol	78 mg

*Dried thyme leaves may be used if fresh thyme is not available.

Pork Chops with Red Cabbage and Apples

4 pork chops (½ inch thick)
1 tablespoon vegetable oil
½ cup chopped red onion
½ head red cabbage
1 large apple, chopped into
  chunks
¼ teaspoon ground black
  pepper
⅛ teaspoon ground cloves

Yield: 4 servings of 1 pork chop with ¼ cup fruit and vegetable mixture

Food Exchanges: 3 lean meats + 1 starch/bread

Brown pork chops in oil in a heavy skillet. Remove chops from pan. Sauté onion in the skillet until clear. Add cabbage chopped into 1-inch pieces and apple. Simmer over medium heat about 5 minutes. Sprinkle pepper and cloves on top. Place chops in the skillet over cabbage. Cover and cook over low heat for 20 minutes, or until chops are tender.

Calories per serving	253
Protein	25 g
Carbohydrate	13 g
Fat	11 g
Sodium	78 mg
Potassium	610 mg
Cholesterol	71 mg

Caraway Pork and Vegetable Stew

1½ pounds lean pork, cubed
1 clove garlic, thinly sliced
½ cup chopped onions
½ cup chopped green pepper
1 cup apple juice
2 teaspoons caraway seeds
½ teaspoon dried thyme leaves
½ teaspoon paprika
1 cup sliced fresh carrots
1 cup fresh green beans, cut
   into bite-size pieces
1 cup sliced fresh mushrooms
24 to 30 cherry tomatoes, cut in
   halves, or 3 whole tomatoes,
   cut into chunks

Yield: 6 ¾-cup servings

Food Exchanges: 3 lean meats +
3 vegetables

Brown pork cubes in a no-stick skillet. Add garlic, onions, green pepper, apple juice, caraway seeds, thyme, and paprika. Cover and cook over medium heat for 15 minutes. Add vegetables. Simmer covered for 15 to 20 minutes or until vegetables are tender. Serve over rice or noodles.*

Calories per serving	269
Protein	27 g
Carbohydrate	14 g
Fat	12 g
Sodium	77 mg
Potassium	736 mg
Cholesterol	78 mg

* Rice or noodles are not included in the nutrient analysis for this recipe. One-third cup of cooked rice or ½ cup of cooked noodles equals 1 starch/bread exchange.

Pork Tenderloin with Pesto

1¼ pounds pork tenderloin, trimmed
¼ cup chopped fresh basil
2 tablespoons chopped fresh parsley
2 tablespoons grated Parmesan cheese
1 clove garlic, minced
1 tablespoon toasted pine nuts
1 teaspoon olive oil

Yield: 4 servings of 3 1-ounce slices

Food Exchanges: 3 medium-fat meats

Cut pork tenderloin in half lengthwise, leaving it attached on one side. Open it like a book. To make the pesto, combine remaining ingredients, except olive oil, in a food processor or blender. Process until blended and spread on pork. Fold the pieces of pork back together. Tie with string or secure with metal skewers. Broil for 6 to 8 minutes on each side until done. Brush with olive oil just before serving.

Calories per serving	239
Protein	26 g
Carbohydrate	0
Fat	14 g
Sodium	106 mg
Potassium	314 mg
Cholesterol	80 mg

Stuffed Cabbage

1 head cabbage
1½ pounds ground veal
½ cup uncooked white rice
1½ cups chopped onion
1 6-ounce can tomato paste
1 egg
½ teaspoon ground black
* pepper*
3 tablespoons vinegar
2 tablespoons brown sugar
1 8-ounce can tomato sauce

Fill a large pot with water and heat until boiling. Immerse cabbage head into water until outer leaves are softened. Continue process until 12 leaves have been removed. Combine veal, rice, ½ cup onion, ¼ cup tomato paste, egg, and pepper in a bowl. Mix thoroughly. Place heaping spoonful on each cabbage leaf. Roll up cabbage leaf around filling. Combine remaining tomato paste with 1 cup water in a large saucepan. Add 1 cup chopped onion, vinegar, and brown sugar. Place cabbage rolls in a pot. Pour tomato sauce over cabbage rolls. Cover and cook for 1½ hours on low heat.

Calories per serving	269
Protein	26 g
Carbohydrate	16 g
Fat	11 g
Sodium	198 mg
Potassium	696 mg
Cholesterol	128 mg

Yield: 6 servings of 1 cabbage roll each

Food Exchanges: 3 lean meats + 1 starch/bread

Veal and Bean Cholent

1 cup dried lima beans
1 cup great northern beans
⅓ cup olive oil
1 onion, finely chopped
2 cloves garlic, minced
2 carrots, peeled and sliced
2 stalks celery, chopped
2 tomatoes, chopped
1 cup dry white wine
4 pounds veal shoulder, cut
   into 2-inch cubes
1 teaspoon paprika
3 bay leaves
½ teaspoon ground black
   pepper
¼ cup chopped fresh parsley
½ teaspoon dried thyme leaves
½ teaspoon dried tarragon
   leaves
1 tablespoon dried oregano
   leaves

In a large bowl, soak beans in cold water overnight. Drain. Heat oil in a large skillet or casserole. Add onion, garlic, carrots, and celery. Sauté until tender. Combine beans, onion mixture, and remaining ingredients in a large saucepan. Add 3 cups water. Cover and bring to a boil over high heat. Put the saucepan in an oven and bake at 250 degrees for 12 hours or overnight.

Calories per serving	293
Protein	24 g
Carbohydrate	18 g
Fat	13 g
Sodium	58 mg
Potassium	591 mg
Cholesterol	65 mg

Yield: 10 2-cup servings

Food Exchanges: 3 lean meats + 1 starch/bread + 1 fat

Pot Roast of Veal

2 cloves garlic, minced
1 small onion, chopped
1 shallot or 2 green onions,
   chopped
1 tablespoon vegetable oil
2 pounds veal shoulder, shank,
   or rump roast
2 cups chicken broth
1 cup dry white wine
20 whole allspice
½ teaspoon ground thyme
4 whole cloves
1 bay leaf
8 whole black peppercorns

Yield: 4 servings of 3 1-ounce
slices

Food Exchanges: 3 medium-fat
meats + 1 vegetable

Sauté garlic, onion, and shallot in oil until transparent in a large casserole. Place veal in pan. Brown on all sides. Add remaining ingredients. Simmer on the range for 1½ hours or until roast is tender.

Calories per serving	274
Protein	24 g
Carbohydrate	5 g
Fat	13 g
Sodium	62 mg
Potassium	353 mg
Cholesterol	81 mg

Italian Easter Pie

4 ounces mild Italian sausage
(links)

4 eggs

1 15-ounce carton part-skim
ricotta cheese

4 ounces prosciutto or cooked
ham, chopped

2 ounces Genoa salami,
chopped

½ cup shredded part-skim
mozzarella cheese

¼ cup grated Parmesan cheese

1 9-inch pastry crust

Fresh parsley

Yield: 8 slices

Food Exchanges: 3 high-fat
meats + 1 starch/bread

Cook sausage in a small amount of water in a covered skillet. Brown sausage on all sides. Beat eggs and ricotta cheese together. Stir in prosciutto, salami, and mozzarella and Parmesan cheeses. Slice sausage and fold into the mixture. Pour the ricotta mixture into a pastry crust. Bake in a 350-degree oven for 45 to 50 minutes, or until a knife inserted in the center comes out clean. Garnish with fresh parsley just before serving.

Calories per slice	338
Protein	20 g
Carbohydrate	24 g
Fat	27 g
Sodium	622 mg
Potassium	203 mg
Cholesterol	201 mg

Note: This recipe contains 400 milligrams or more of sodium per serving.

This recipe is high in saturated fat, cholesterol, and calories. It should be reserved for very special occasions only.

Beef Stew with Acorn Squash

3½ pounds boneless lean beef
  roast
2 large onions, chopped
1½ cups apple juice
2½ cups water
1 cinnamon stick or ½
  teaspoon of ground
  cinnamon
2 large acorn squash (3
  pounds)
¼ cup raisins

Yield: 8 1-cup servings

Food Exchanges: 4 lean meats +
1 starch/bread

Cut beef roast into 1-inch pieces. Brown in a no-stick skillet or casserole with onions. Stir in apple juice, water, and cinnamon. Cover and cook over low heat about 2 hours, or until meat is tender when pierced with a fork. Meanwhile, peel squash and remove seeds. Cut into 1-inch cubes. When meat is tender, add squash and raisins. Cover and simmer about 15 minutes longer until squash is tender.

Calories per serving	295
Protein	29 g
Carbohydrate	19 g
Fat	9 g
Sodium	59 mg
Potassium	800 mg
Cholesterol	82 mg

Baked Beef Brisket

4 pounds boneless beef brisket
½ teaspoon ground black
  pepper
1 clove garlic, minced
3 large onions, sliced

Trim fat off beef brisket and place in a roasting pan. Sprinkle on pepper, garlic, and onions. Bake in a 350-degree oven for 1 hour. Add 1 cup water to the roasting pan. Cover with foil. Continue roasting in a 300-degree oven for 2 hours. Carve brisket into thin slices.

Yield: 10 servings of 3 1-ounce
slices

Food Exchanges: 3 lean meats

Calories per serving	164
Protein	22 g
Carbohydrate	2 g
Fat	7 g
Sodium	46 mg
Potassium	306 mg
Cholesterol	66 mg

Beefy Split Pea Stew

½ pound boneless beef round
steak
½ cup chopped onion
3 cups water
½ cup dried split peas
2 large carrots, sliced
2 white potatoes, cubed
2 sweet potatoes, cubed
2 tablespoons chopped fresh
parsley or 1 tablespoon dried
parsley flakes
½ teaspoon salt
½ teaspoon dried thyme leaves
⅛ teaspoon ground nutmeg
Pinch black pepper
2 cups chopped fresh spinach

Cut steak into cubes. Brown in a no-stick skillet. Add onion and sauté until browned. Add remaining ingredients, except spinach. Cook over low heat for 50 to 55 minutes, or until meat and potatoes are tender. Add spinach. Turn off heat and let steam for 5 minutes before serving.

Calories per serving	301
Protein	22 g
Carbohydrate	47 g
Fat	4 g
Sodium	331 mg
Potassium	986 mg
Cholesterol	41 mg

Yield: 4 ⅔-cup servings

Food Exchanges: 2 lean meats +
3 starch/breads

Steak Diane

2½ pounds beef flank steak or
  beef tenderloin
1 medium onion
½ cup red wine
1 teaspoon prepared mustard
2 to 4 tablespoons brandy
Brandy for flaming

Cut flank steak into diagonal slices. Slice onion thin and sauté in wine. Add mustard and brandy. Cook until onion is tender. Add steak slices and cook for 3 to 5 minutes. Bring the skillet to the table. Pour about 1 tablespoon brandy over beef slices. Pour another tablespoon brandy into a large serving spoon. Heat brandy in the spoon using a candle or sterno. When brandy is hot, ignite and pour over meat and brandy in the skillet. Stir to blend flavors just before serving.

Yield: 6 servings of 8 ½-ounce slices

Calories per serving	207
Protein	27 g
Carbohydrate	4 g
Fat	5 g
Sodium	78 mg
Potassium	344 mg
Cholesterol	82 mg

Food Exchanges: 4 lean meats

Cardamom Pot Roast

2 to 2½ pounds beef pot roast
½ cup wine vinegar
½ cup rose wine
½ cup chopped onion
2 teaspoons ground cardamom
2 bay leaves
2 whole peppercorns
8 whole cloves
8 whole allspice

Brown pot roast in a no-stick skillet. Place in a casserole or roasting pan. Combine remaining ingredients. Pour over roast. Cover and cook in a 325-degree oven about 1 hour.

Calories per serving	186
Protein	27 g
Carbohydrate	3 g
Fat	5 g
Sodium	67 mg
Potassium	358 mg
Cholesterol	82 mg

Yield: 6 servings of 4 1-ounce slices

Food Exchanges: 4 lean meats

Beef Roulade

2 pounds beef flank steak
½ cup chopped carrots
½ cup chopped green onion
½ cup chopped celery
1 clove garlic, minced
¼ cup chopped fresh parsley
½ teaspoon dried marjoram
   leaves
1 teaspoon dried thyme leaves
¼ teaspoon ground black
   pepper
Tomato juice (optional)

Place flank steak on a flat surface and cut in half, starting on the thick side. Lay steak flat like a book, leaving one end *not* cut. Combine remaining ingredients in a mixing bowl. Spread over meat and roll up lengthwise. Keep roll closed by tying with string or fastening with metal meat skewers. Bake in a 375-degree oven for 1 hour. Baste with tomato juice, if desired.

Calories per serving	170
Protein	27 g
Carbohydrate	2 g
Fat	5 g
Sodium	81 mg
Potassium	380 mg
Cholesterol	82 mg

Yield: 6 servings of 4 1-ounce slices

Food Exchanges: 4 lean meats

Grapefruit Chicken and Vegetables

*1 3-pound chicken, cut into
serving pieces*
1 tablespoon vegetable oil
4 carrots, pared and sliced
1 small onion, thinly sliced
2 stalks celery, chopped
*1 tablespoon minced fresh
ginger root*
1 teaspoon ground coriander
*½ teaspoon ground white
pepper*
2 grapefruit
*2 tablespoons chopped fresh
parsley*

Yield: 6 3-ounce servings

Food Exchanges: 3 lean meats +
1 fruit

Remove skin from chicken and brown in oil in a large skillet or deep kettle. Add carrots, onion, celery, ginger root, coriander, and pepper. Peel and section grapefruit over bowl to catch juice. Add juice and sections from one grapefruit to chicken. Cover and cook over medium heat for 40 to 50 minutes, or until chicken is tender. Top with reserved grapefruit sections and parsley just before serving.

Calories per serving	200
Protein	21 g
Carbohydrate	13 g
Fat	8 g
Sodium	81 mg
Potassium	485 mg
Cholesterol	55 mg

Easy Chicken Stew

4 chicken legs and thighs
4 medium potatoes
4 carrots, sliced
1 small onion, sliced

Place chicken in a baking dish or on aluminum foil. Quarter potato and place around chicken. Add carrots and onion. Cover the baking dish or seal the foil. Bake in a 350-degree oven for 50 minutes or until chicken is tender.

Yield: 4 servings

Food Exchanges: 3 lean meats +
2 starches/breads + 1 vegetable

Calories per serving	336
Protein	21 g
Carbohydrate	42 g
Fat	10 g
Sodium	94 mg
Potassium	1,197 mg
Cholesterol	58 mg

Chicken Breasts Scallopini

2 whole chicken breasts, split

1 tablespoon vegetable or olive oil

½ cup thinly sliced onion

2 cloves garlic, minced

½ cup sliced mushrooms

½ cup tomato sauce

¼ cup white wine or apple juice

½ teaspoon dried oregano leaves

½ teaspoon dried thyme leaves

2 tablespoons grated Parmesan cheese

Sauté chicken breasts in oil until browned. Add onion, garlic, and mushrooms. Simmer for 5 minutes until onion is tender. Stir in tomato sauce, wine, oregano, and thyme. Cover the skillet and simmer for 10 minutes. Sprinkle cheese on top just before serving.

Calories per serving	152
Protein	13 g
Carbohydrate	6 g
Fat	7 g
Sodium	241 mg
Potassium	298 mg
Cholesterol	33 mg

Yield: 4 servings of ½ chicken breast

Food Exchanges: 2 lean meats + 1 vegetable

Moroccan Chicken

1 3-pound chicken, cut into serving pieces, or 4 split chicken breasts

8 dried figs, snipped

1 8-ounce can tomato sauce

½ cup chopped onion

2 cloves garlic, minced

¼ cup white wine or apple juice

2 bay leaves

½ teaspoon ground allspice

1 teaspoon dried thyme leaves

½ cup chopped green pepper (optional)

2 tablespoons toasted sesame seeds or slivered almonds

Yield: 6 3-ounce servings

Food Exchanges: 3 lean meats + 1 fruit + 1 vegetable

Skin chicken. Place in a pot or heavy skillet. Add remaining ingredients, except sesame seeds or almonds. Cover and cook in a slow cooker or on low heat for 2½ hours to 3 hours, or until chicken is tender. For faster cooking, bring to a boil on top of the range, reduce heat to low, and cook for 25 to 30 minutes. Sprinkle sesame seeds or almonds on top just before serving.

Calories per serving	241
Protein	22 g
Carbohydrate	22 g
Fat	7 g
Sodium	270 mg
Potassium	553 mg
Cholesterol	55 mg

Rosemary Chicken Dijon

1 pound boneless chicken
   breasts
1 tablespoon vegetable oil
2 shallots or green onions,
   thinly sliced
2 cloves garlic, minced
1 tablespoon Dijon mustard
½ teaspoon ground rosemary
½ cup chicken broth
4 large fresh mushrooms,
   sliced
1 tablespoon cornstarch
2 tablespoons chopped
   pimento

Yield: 4 servings of ½ chicken
breast

Food Exchanges: 3 lean meats +
1 vegetable

Sauté chicken breasts in oil until browned on all sides. Add shallots and garlic. Simmer until shallots are tender. Stir in mustard, rosemary, and broth. Top with mushrooms. Simmer for 10 minutes, or until chicken is tender. Dissolve cornstarch in a small amount of cold water. Stir into the mixture. Cook over medium heat until thickened. Top with pimento just before serving on rice.*

Calories per serving	192
Protein	23 g
Carbohydrate	3 g
Fat	9 g
Sodium	101 mg
Potassium	237 mg
Cholesterol	62 mg

* Rice is not included in the nutrient analysis for this recipe. One-third cup of cooked rice equals 1 starch/bread exchange.

Chicken with Raspberry Sauce

3 whole chicken breasts,
skinned
1 tablespoon olive oil
1 clove garlic, minced
1 small onion, finely chopped
2 tablespoons raspberry* or
cider vinegar
¼ cup plain yogurt
15 to 20 fresh raspberries for
garnish

Cut each chicken breast in half and flatten with a meat mallet. Combine oil, garlic, and onion in a skillet. Add chicken breasts. Sauté over medium heat just until browned. Reduce heat to low, cover, and simmer for 15 minutes or until chicken is tender. Add water if needed to prevent sticking. Remove chicken breasts. Add vinegar and yogurt to the skillet and stir until blended. DO NOT BOIL SAUCE. Serve chicken breasts with sauce poured over them. Garnish with raspberries.

Calories per serving	193
Protein	25 g
Carbohydrate	2 g
Fat	8 g
Sodium	66 mg
Potassium	251 mg
Cholesterol	70 mg

Yield: 6 servings of ½ chicken breast

Food Exchanges: 3 lean meats

*Available in gourmet or specialty food stores.

Chicken with Orange Dill Sauce

1 whole chicken breast, cut in
half
1 green onion, minced
1 teaspoon sesame seeds
1 teaspoon grated orange rind
¼ teaspoon dried dill weed
2 teaspoons vegetable oil
1 teaspoon cornstarch
¼ cup orange juice

Steam chicken until tender, about 15 to 20 minutes. Make sauce by combining onion, sesame seeds, orange rind, and dill in a small saucepan or skillet with vegetable oil. Cook until onion is tender. Dissolve cornstarch in orange juice. Stir into onion mixture. Cook over medium heat until thickened. Pour sauce over chicken breast just before serving.

Yield: 2 servings of ½ chicken
breast

Food Exchanges: 4 lean meats

Calories per serving	235
Protein	30 g
Carbohydrate	5 g
Fat	10 g
Sodium	10 mg
Potassium	307 mg
Cholesterol	83 mg

Chicken Breasts in Pimento Sauce

2 whole chicken breasts,
deboned
1 tablespoon vegetable oil
2 green onions, chopped
1 cup sliced mushrooms
2 ounces low-fat cheese, thinly
sliced
1 4-ounce jar pimento strips
Fresh chopped parsley

Split chicken breasts. Sauté in oil until browned. Set aside. Add onions and mushrooms to oil. Simmer until onions are soft. Place mushroom mixture in the bottom of a baking dish. Arrange chicken breasts over the mixture. Lay cheese slices over chicken. Sprinkle pimento on top. Cover and bake in a 350-degree oven for 20 minutes, or until tender. Garnish with parsley just before serving.

Yield: 4 servings of ½ chicken
breast

Food Exchanges: 4 lean meats

Calories per serving	225
Protein	29 g
Carbohydrate	1 g
Fat	12 g
Sodium	121 mg
Potassium	273 mg
Cholesterol	70 mg

Chicken Breasts Florentine

2 whole chicken breasts,
  deboned
1 10-ounce package frozen
  spinach
½ cup chopped onion
¼ teaspoon ground nutmeg
⅓ cup grated Swiss cheese
1 tablespoon olive oil
1 shallot, chopped
8 ounces fresh mushrooms,
  thinly sliced
½ cup chicken broth
2 tablespoons finely chopped
  fresh basil or 1 teaspoon
  dried basil leaves

Yield: 4 servings of ½ chicken
breast

Food Exchanges: 4 lean meats

Split chicken breasts and flatten with a meat mallet. Simmer spinach, onion, and nutmeg together in a no-stick skillet. Cool. Place equal amounts of spinach mixture on each breast. Roll up chicken around spinach and cheese. Steam over hot water in a saucepan for 15 to 20 minutes until chicken is tender. Prepare mushrooms sauce by combining oil, shallots, and mushrooms in a skillet. Sauté until mushrooms are tender. Add chicken broth and simmer. When ready to serve, pour sauce over chicken and sprinkle basil on top.

Calories per serving	229
Protein	28 g
Carbohydrate	5 g
Fat	11 g
Sodium	159 mg
Potassium	595 mg
Cholesterol	69 mg

Chicken with Fruit and Cashews

4 whole chicken breasts, cut into 1-inch pieces
1 tablespoon vegetable oil
2 to 4 teaspoons curry powder
12 canned or fresh apricot halves
1½ cups green seedless grapes
24 to 30 cherry tomatoes, cut in half
¼ cup unsalted roasted cashew nuts
Lemon slices
Plain low-fat yogurt

Sauté chicken in oil until tender. Stir in curry powder. Add remaining ingredients, except lemon slices and yogurt. Stir lightly until chicken is well done. Spoon onto serving platter. Garnish with lemon slices and top with yogurt.

Calories per serving	246
Protein	24 g
Carbohydrate	14 g
Fat	11 g
Sodium	73 mg
Potassium	435 mg
Cholesterol	62 mg

Yield: 8 ½-cup servings

Food Exchanges: 3 lean meats + 1 fruit

Baked Chicken with Matzo Stuffing

1 tablespoon olive oil
1 onion, chopped
2 stalks celery, chopped
1 tablespoon chopped parsley
1 clove garlic, minced
1 teaspoon dried sage leaves
½ teaspoon dried rosemary
* leaves*
4 6½-inch squares matzo
¼ cup chicken stock or water
1 3-pound chicken

Yield: 6 servings of 3 ounces chicken and ½ cup stuffing

Food Exchanges: 2 medium-fat meats + 1½ starches/breads + 1 fat

Combine oil, onion, celery, parsley, garlic, sage, and rosemary in a skillet. Sauté until onion is tender, about 10 minutes. Fill a large baking dish with water. Add matzo and soak until softened. Drain well. Gently squeeze out excess water. Tear matzo into ¼-inch pieces. Add matzo to onion mixture. Stir in chicken stock to moisten stuffing. Spoon stuffing into chicken. Bake in a 350-degree oven for 45 to 50 minutes.

Calories per serving	296
Protein	17 g
Carbohydrate	21 g
Fat	16 g
Sodium	249 mg
Potassium	283 mg
Cholesterol	44 mg

Chicken Curry Stew

2 whole chicken breasts, cut in
 half
1 small onion, chopped
2 cloves garlic, minced
6 whole cloves
9 whole black peppercorns
4 whole cardamom pods
1 teaspoon ground coriander
¼ teaspoon ground cumin
1 tablespoon minced fresh
 gingerroot
¼ teaspoon ground turmeric
⅛ teaspoon ground nutmeg
½ cup chicken broth
Chopped fresh coriander

Cut chicken breasts into bite-size pieces. Brown chicken in a no-stick skillet with onion and garlic. Add remaining ingredients, except fresh coriander. Simmer for 40 minutes or until tender. Sprinkle coriander on top and serve over rice with accompaniments of raisins, coconut, chopped onion, and tomatoes.*

Calories per serving	154
Protein	23 g
Carbohydrate	2 g
Fat	6 g
Sodium	72 mg
Potassium	280 mg
Cholesterol	83 mg

Yield: 4 ½-cup servings

Food Exchanges: 3 lean meats

*Rice and accompaniments are not included in the nutrient analysis for this recipe. One-third cup of cooked rice equals 1 starch/bread exchange. Use small amounts of accompaniments as allowed in your individual meal plan.

Herbed Chicken with Vegetables

1 3-pound chicken, cut into
serving pieces
¼ teaspoon ground white
pepper
1 teaspoon paprika
½ teaspoon dried thyme leaves
½ teaspoon dried basil leaves
2 cloves garlic, minced
2 large onions, sliced
1 bay leaf
4 carrots, cut into 1-inch pieces
8 small potatoes
1 cup apple juice

Yield: 6 servings of ⅙ chicken
and ½ cup vegetables

Food Exchanges: 3 lean meats +
1 starch/bread + 2 vegetables

Rub chicken with pepper and paprika. Place chicken pieces in a baking pan. Sprinkle on thyme and basil. Add remaining ingredients to the baking pan. Cover and bake in a 350-degree oven about 50 minutes or until chicken is tender.

Calories per serving	276
Protein	23 g
Carbohydrate	27 g
Fat	5 g
Sodium	76 mg
Potassium	766 mg
Cholesterol	55 mg

Cornish Hen with Wild Rice Stuffing

2 Cornish hens
1 orange
2 teaspoons margarine
1 green onion
½ apple, finely chopped
2 tablespoons raisins
1 tablespoon brandy or apple
  juice
⅔ cup cooked wild rice
¼ teaspoon dried thyme leaves
2 tablespoons orange juice
  concentrate

Yield: 4 servings of ½ hen with
½ cup stuffing

Food Exchanges: 3 lean meats +
1 starch/bread + ½ fruit + 1 fat

Wash hens and pat dry. Grate orange and rub outer surface of hens with grated peel. Melt margarine in a skillet. Add onion and apple. Sauté until onion is tender. Plump raisins in brandy. Combine onion mixture, raisins, rice, and thyme in a bowl. Mix well. Stuff hens. Bake in a 350-degree oven for 35 to 40 minutes. Baste with orange juice concentrate while baking.

Calories per serving	311
Protein	22 g
Carbohydrate	25 g
Fat	13 g
Sodium	148 mg
Potassium	428 mg
Cholesterol	66 mg

Turkey Tacos

2 cups cooked, diced turkey
1 small onion, minced
1 clove garlic, minced
1 teaspoon cumin seeds
6 corn tortillas
1 cup shredded lettuce
1 ripe tomato, diced
3 tablespoons taco sauce
½ cup grated cheddar cheese

Yield: 6 servings of 1 taco

Food Exchanges: 2 lean meats +
1 starch/bread

Combine turkey, onion, garlic, and cumin seeds in a no-stick skillet. Simmer until onion is tender. Spoon turkey mixture into tortillas. Top with lettuce, tomato, taco sauce, and cheese.

Calories per serving	195
Protein	18 g
Carbohydrate	17 g
Fat	6 g
Sodium	168 mg
Potassium	275 mg
Cholesterol	46 mg

Turkey Piccata

1 pound fresh or frozen turkey
   breast slices
1 teaspoon vegetable oil
¼ cup white wine or apple
   juice
½ cup sliced fresh mushrooms
2 tablespoons lemon juice
2 tablespoons chopped fresh
   parsley
2 tablespoons capers
Lemon slices

Sauté turkey with oil in skillet over medium heat until browned. Add wine, mushrooms, lemon juice, and parsley. Cook until turkey is tender. Add capers. Serve with lemon slices.

Calories per serving	149
Protein	21 g
Carbohydrate	2 g
Fat	5 g
Sodium	51 mg
Potassium	269 mg
Cholesterol	54 mg

Yield: 4 servings of 1 3-ounce slice

Food Exchanges: 3 lean meats

Rabbit Marengo

1 rabbit (about 2 pounds), cut
   up*
1 clove garlic, minced
½ teaspoon dried thyme leaves
½ teaspoon dried basil leaves
1 teaspoon dried parsley leaves
4 whole tomatoes or 1 16-ounce
   can tomatoes
½ cup white wine
¼ pound fresh mushrooms,
   sliced

Combine rabbit pieces, garlic, thyme, basil, parsley, and tomatoes in a large saucepan. Stir in wine. Bring to a boil, reduce heat, cover, and simmer about 40 minutes until rabbit is tender. Stir in mushrooms during last 10 minutes of cooking.

Calories per serving	253
Protein	28 g
Carbohydrate	8 g
Fat	9 g
Sodium	43 mg
Potassium	699 mg
Cholesterol	59 mg

Yield: 4 servings of 4 ounces

Food Exchanges: 4 lean meats +
1 vegetable

*Chicken may be substituted.

Pastitsio

7 ounces uncooked elbow
  macaroni
½ cup skim milk
¼ cup grated Parmesan cheese
2 egg whites
1 pound ground turkey or 1
  cup cooked chopped turkey
  pieces
½ cup chopped onion
1 clove garlic, minced
8 ounces tomato sauce (1 cup)
2 teaspoons ground cinnamon
¼ teaspoon nutmeg
2 tablespoons grated Parmesan
  cheese
Fresh grated nutmeg (optional)

Yield: 6 servings

Food Exchanges: 2 lean meats +
1½ starches/breads

Cook macaroni according to package directions. Drain. Combine macaroni, milk, ¼ cup cheese, and egg white. Place half of mixture in an oiled casserole. Make the sauce by combining turkey, onion, garlic, tomato sauce, cinnamon, and nutmeg in a skillet. Cook until onion is tender. Spoon mixture over macaroni layer. Top with remaining macaroni. Sprinkle 2 tablespoons cheese on top. Bake in a 350-degree oven for 35 to 40 minutes. Sprinkle fresh grated nutmeg on top before serving, if desired

Calories per serving	214
Protein	16 g
Carbohydrate	27 g
Fat	5 g
Sodium	368 mg
Potassium	369 mg
Cholesterol	68 mg

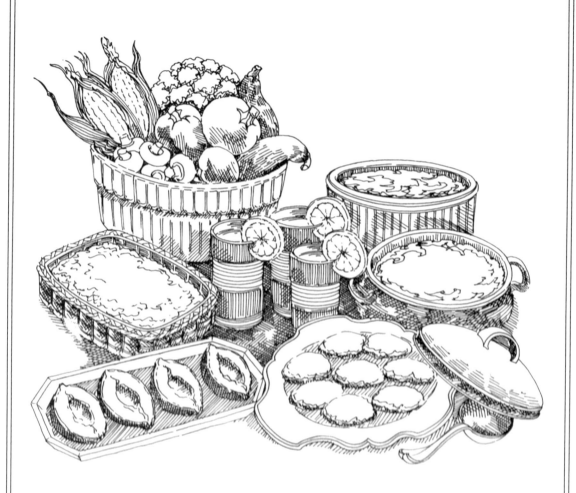

6

Vegetarian
Entrées

Crustless Broccoli Quiche

5 eggs
1 small onion, finely chopped
½ teaspoon ground nutmeg
1 10-ounce package frozen
  chopped broccoli, defrosted
8 ounces part-skim mozzarella
  cheese, grated

Combine all ingredients in a mixing bowl. Beat well. Pour into a lightly oiled 8-inch pie plate. Bake in a 350-degree oven for 25 to 30 minutes, or until a knife inserted into the center comes out clean. Serve hot.

Calories per serving	185
Protein	17 g
Carbohydrate	4 g
Fat	12 g
Sodium	238 mg
Potassium	181 mg
Cholesterol	250 mg

Yield: 6 servings

Food Exchanges: 2 medium-fat meats + 1 vegetable + 1 fat

Note: This recipe contains more than ½ egg per serving.

Noodle Kugel with Vegetables

1 pound wide egg noodles
1 tablespoon vegetable oil
2 large onions, minced
1 cup sliced fresh mushrooms
1 teaspoon dried thyme leaves
1 teaspoon paprika
4 large eggs, beaten
¼ cup chopped cilantro or
  parsley
2 large carrots, grated
2 small zucchini, grated

Prepare noodles according to package directions. Drain. Heat oil in a skillet. Sauté onions and mushrooms in the skillet with thyme and paprika until onions are tender. Combine mushroom mixture, noodles, and remaining ingredients. Pour into a lightly oiled baking dish. Bake in a 350-degree oven for 45 to 50 minutes or until mixture is set (when a knife inserted in the center comes out clean).

Yield: 8 servings

Food Exchanges: 1 starch/bread + 1 fat + 1 vegetable

Calories per serving	149
Protein	6 g
Carbohydrate	20 g
Fat	5 g
Sodium	40 mg
Potassium	229 mg
Cholesterol	129 mg

Split Peas Pizza

2 ½ cups cooked brown rice
1 egg
¾ cup grated cheddar cheese
¾ cup cooked, mashed split
  peas
1 8-ounce can tomato paste
2 teaspoons dried oregano
  leaves
2 teaspoons dried thyme leaves
½ teaspoon dried basil leaves
¼ cup water
1 cup shredded part-skim
  mozzarella cheese

Yield: 8 servings

Food Exchanges: 1 medium-fat
meat + 1½ starches/breads

To make crust, mix rice, egg, and cheddar cheese together with a fork. Pat mixture into a lightly oiled 10-inch pie pan or pizza pan. Bake in a 450-degree oven for 15 minutes. To make the topping, combine peas, tomato paste, oregano, thyme, basil, and water. Spread over crust. Sprinkle on mozzarella cheese. Bake in a 450-degree oven for 10 minutes.

Calories per serving	198
Protein	11 g
Carbohydrate	23 g
Fat	7 g
Sodium	327 mg
Potassium	263 mg
Cholesterol	54 mg

Spinach Matzo Kugel

3 matzo crackers
1 tablespoon vegetable oil
1 ½ cups sliced fresh mushrooms
½ cup chopped onion
6 eggs
1 tablespoon lemon juice
1 teaspoon grated lemon peel
1 10-ounce package frozen chopped spinach, thawed and drained
1 cup low-fat cottage cheese
1 2-ounce jar chopped pimento, drained

Soak crackers in warm water just until softened. Squeeze out extra water. Combine oil, mushrooms, and onion in a skillet. Sauté until onion is tender. Beat eggs, lemon juice, and lemon peel together in a large mixing bowl. Add onion mixture, spinach, cottage cheese, and pimento. Place one matzo cracker on the bottom of a lightly oiled 8-inch baking pan. Cut another matzo cracker into four strips and place them around the sides of the baking pan. Pour in about half of egg mixture. Place the other matzo cracker on top of the vegetable-egg mixture. Pour on remaining mixture. Bake in a 350-degree oven for 25 to 30 minutes or until a knife inserted in the center comes out clean.

Calories per serving	276
Protein	17 g
Carbohydrate	21 g
Fat	13 g
Sodium	363 mg
Potassium	451 mg
Cholesterol	369 mg

Yield: 6 servings

Food Exchanges: 2 medium-fat meats + 1 starch/bread + 1 fat

Note: This recipe contains more than ½ egg and 300 milligrams of cholesterol per serving.

Stuffed Acorn Squash

2 acorn squash
2 cooking apples, diced
1 tablespoon chopped onion
2 tablespoons chopped fresh
  parsley
½ teaspoon ground cinnamon
Dash nutmeg for each serving

Yield: 4 servings of ½ squash

Food Exchanges: 1 starch/bread
+ ½ fruit

Cut squash in half and scrape out seeds. Arrange squash in a baking dish. Combine apples, onion, parsley, and cinnamon. Divide mixture and fill each squash. Cover with foil or parchment paper. Bake in a 400-degree oven for 40 to 50 minutes, or until squash is fork-tender. Sprinkle on nutmeg just before serving.

Calories per serving	104
Protein	2 g
Carbohydrate	26 g
Fat	0
Sodium	1 mg
Potassium	544 mg
Cholesterol	0

Lentil-Potato Patties

½ cup chopped onion
1 tablespoon vegetable oil
2 cups cooked lentils, puréed
2 cups mashed potatoes
1 teaspoon ground sage
½ teaspoon salt
¼ teaspoon ground black
  pepper

Yield: 6 servings of 2 patties

Food Exchanges: 1 starch/bread
+ 1 fat

Sauté onion in oil until tender. Combine lentils, potatoes, sage, salt, pepper, and onion. Mix well. Form into 12 patties. Bake in a 400-degree oven for 15 to 20 minutes or sauté in a no-stick pan for 5 minutes on each side.

Calories per serving	127
Protein	6 g
Carbohydrate	18 g
Fat	4 g
Sodium	112 mg
Potassium	277 mg
Cholesterol	0

Beans and Rice Casserole

*1 15-ounce can (2 cups) red
  kidney beans*
1 cup cooked brown rice
*1 ½ teaspoons dried thyme
  leaves*
¼ cup chopped onions
1 teaspoon vegetable oil
½ cup grated cheddar cheese

Yield: 4 1-cup servings

Food Exchanges: 1 lean meat +
3 starches/breads

Combine beans, rice, and thyme. Sauté onions in oil until tender. Add to bean mixture. Pour into an oiled casserole dish. Bake in a 350-degree oven for 20 to 30 minutes. Sprinkle on cheese. Return to oven for 5 minutes to melt cheese.

Calories per serving	294
Protein	16 g
Carbohydrate	44 g
Fat	7 g
Sodium	242 mg
Potassium	534 mg
Cholesterol	15 mg

Lentil Cutlets

*5 ounces dried lentils, soaked
  overnight*
2 tablespoons vegetable oil
1 large onion, finely chopped
1 tablespoon flour
1 to 2 teaspoons curry powder
*1 tablespoon plain low-fat
  yogurt*
1 teaspoon salt
Oil for frying
*Fresh chopped cilantro leaves
  or parsley*

Yield: 6 servings of 1 cutlet each

Food Exchanges: 1 lean meat +
1 starch/bread + 2 fats

Drain and finely grind lentils. Sauté 2 tablespoons oil and onion together in a skillet. Add flour and curry powder and cook for 3 minutes. Remove from heat and cool. Add ground lentils, yogurt, and salt. Mix well and form into 6 cutlets. Heat oil for frying. Cook cutlets until golden brown. Drain. Serve hot with chopped cilantro leaves.

Calories per serving	278
Protein	8 g
Carbohydrate	22 g
Fat	15 g
Sodium	329 mg
Potassium	287 mg
Cholesterol	14 mg

Beans and Pasta

2 cups canned great northern
  beans
1 small onion, chopped
1 28-ounce can plum tomatoes,
  chopped
1½ cups uncooked rigatoni or
  macaroni shells
1 cup water
1 teaspoon dried rosemary
  leaves
Chopped fresh parsley
1 teaspoon grated Parmesan
  cheese

Combine all ingredients, except parsley and Parmesan cheese, in a saucepan. Cook over a low heat until pasta is tender. Sprinkle on parsley and cheese.

Calories per serving	151
Protein	5 g
Carbohydrate	31 g
Fat	1 g
Sodium	159 mg
Potassium	359 mg
Cholesterol	0

Yield: 4 1-cup servings

Food Exchanges: 2 starches/breads

7

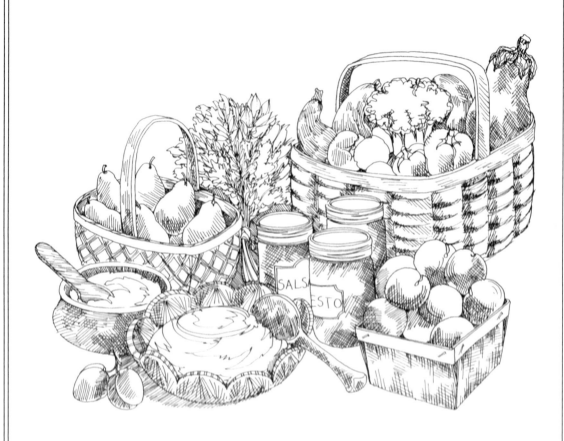

Sauces, Relishes, and Snacks

Crème Fraîche

1 cup heavy cream
2 tablespoons plain low-fat
   yogurt

Mix cream and yogurt in a bowl. Cover and stand at room temperature for 24 hours. Chill until needed. Whip like whipped cream just before serving.* Use within 2 weeks.

Calories per tablespoon serving	46
Protein	0
Carbohydrate	0
Fat	5 g
Sodium	7 mg
Potassium	15 mg
Cholesterol	21 mg

Yield: 16 1-tablespoon servings
or 1 cup

Food Exchange: 1 fat

* May be sweetened with a sugar substitute to use as a dessert topping.

Plum Sauce for Fruit

3 cups sliced fresh plums
½ cup water
1 cinnamon stick
4 packets sugar substitute

Cook plums in water with cinnamon stick until soft. Remove cinnamon. Then purée in a blender or food processor. Cool. Add sugar substitute. Chill. Serve over fresh fruit.

Calories per ½ cup	49
Protein	0
Carbohydrate	12 g
Fat	0
Sodium	0
Potassium	137 mg
Cholesterol	0

Yield: 5 ½-cup servings or
2½ cups sauce

Food Exchange: 1 fruit

Rhubarb Sauce

1 pound fresh rhubarb
4 packets sugar substitute

Cut rhubarb into 1-inch pieces and cook until soft and tender. Mash with a spoon. Cool thoroughly. Stir in sugar substitute. Serve as a spread on toast or biscuits, or as a sauce on fruit salad.

Calories per 2 tablespoons 5
Protein	0
Carbohydrate	1 g
Fat	0
Sodium	0
Potassium	77 mg
Cholesterol	0

Yield: 16 2-tablespoon servings or 2 cups

Food Exchange: Free

Caesar Salad Dressing

2 tablespoons lemon juice
2 tablespoons cider vinegar
⅛ teaspoon dry mustard
1 clove garlic
¼ cup olive oil
1 egg
2 tablespoons grated Parmesan
  cheese

Blend all ingredients together until smooth. Serve over romaine lettuce.

Calories per serving	62
Protein	2 g
Carbohydrate	0
Fat	6 g
Sodium	26 mg
Potassium	16 mg
Cholesterol	48 mg

Yield: 5 2-tablespoon servings or ⅔ cup dressing

Food Exchange: 1 fat

Homemade Mincemeat

2 pounds apples, cored and
   chopped
½ cup brown sugar
½ pound ground beef
1 cup raisins or currants
½ cup chopped citron
½ cup chopped orange peel
½ cup chopped lemon peel
½ teaspoon ground cinnamon
¼ teaspoon ground allspice
¼ teaspoon ground mace or
   nutmeg
2 tablespoons brandy or 2
   teaspoons brandy extract

Yield: 4 cups

Food Exchanges: Mincemeat is
an ingredient in other recipes.
Check those recipes for the exchange values.

Combine all ingredients in a saucepan. Cover and
simmer for 2 hours, stirring frequently. Let cool and
use for mincemeat pie, cookies, or cake, or freeze
until needed.

Calories per ½ cup	226
Protein	6 g
Carbohydrate	44 g
Fat	5 g
Sodium	19 mg
Potassium	343 mg
Cholesterol	21 mg

Pesto

2 cups fresh basil leaves, stems
   removed
¼ cup olive oil
2 tablespoons toasted pine nuts
2 garlic cloves, peeled
¼ cup grated Parmesan cheese

Yield: 32 1-tablespoon servings
or 2 cups

Food Exchange: ½ fat

Combine all ingredients in a food processor. Blend
until well mixed. Serve with pasta, scrambled eggs,
potatoes, or poached fish. May be frozen.

Calories per tablespoon	21
Protein	0
Carbohydrate	0
Fat	2 g
Sodium	12 mg
Potassium	2 mg
Cholesterol	0

Parmigiana Sauce

2 pounds fresh tomatoes
1 clove garlic, minced
1 medium onion, thinly sliced
¼ cup olive oil
¼ cup chopped fresh basil
1 sprig fresh parsley, chopped
½ teaspoon salt (optional)

Chop tomatoes and place in a food processor. Sauté garlic and onion in oil until softened. Add basil, parsley, and salt (optional). Pour into a food processor and purée until smooth. Cook over medium heat for 20 minutes. Cool. Use in parmigiana, ravioli, and pasta dishes.

Yield: 8 ¼-cup servings or 2 cups

Food Exchanges: 1 vegetable + 1 fat

Calories per ¼ cup	84
Protein	1 g
Carbohydrate	5 g
Fat	7 g
Sodium	4 mg
Potassium	243 mg
Cholesterol	0

Dill Sauce for Fish

¼ cup low-fat cottage cheese
¼ cup plain low-fat yogurt
½ teaspoon ground mustard
1 tablespoon finely chopped
   onion
1 tablespoon minced fresh
   parsley flakes or 1 teaspoon
   dried parsley flakes
1 tablespoon minced fresh dill
   weed or 1 teaspoon dried dill
   weed

Purée all ingredients in a blender or food processor. Chill to blend flavors. Serve with fish.

Calories per tablespoon	9
Protein	1 g
Carbohydrate	1 g
Fat	0
Sodium	34 mg
Potassium	25 mg
Cholesterol	1 mg

Yield: 8 1-tablespoon servings
or ½ cup sauce

Food Exchange: Free

Marinade for Seafood

2 tablespoons olive oil
2 tablespoons lemon or lime
  juice
1 clove garlic, chopped
½ teaspoon grated lemon peel
1 tablespoon minced fresh
  parsley
½ teaspoon dried basil, dill, or
  thyme

Yield: ¼ cup

Food Exchange: This recipe is for use with a variety of other foods. Marinating in this liquid will increase the fat content of other foods by 1 gram per ounce and will increase calories by 9 calories per ounce.

Combine ingredients in a blender. Purée until garlic is finely minced. Let stand for 1 hour or overnight before using on fish, lobster, scallops, or shrimp.

Calories per ¼ cup	251
Protein	0
Carbohydrate	4 g
Fat	27 g
Sodium	1 mg
Potassium	54 mg
Cholesterol	0

Mustard Dill Sauce for Fish

2 teaspoons prepared mustard
1 teaspoon minced green onion
1 teaspoon olive oil
¼ teaspoon dried dill weed
1 tablespoon lemon juice

Yield: Enough sauce for 1
pound of fish fillets

Food Exchange: Free when used
on a 3- to 4-ounce serving of fish.

Combine all ingredients in a small bowl. Coat fish
with sauce before broiling or baking.

Calories per tablespoon	51
Protein	0
Carbohydrate	2 g
Fat	5 g
Sodium	126 mg
Potassium	38 mg
Cholesterol	0

Jicama Cucumber Relish

2 cups peeled and shredded
   jicama* (about ½ pound)
2 cups seeded and shredded
   unpeeled cucumber
¼ cup chopped pimento
1 teaspoon salt
1 cup vinegar
1 teaspoon celery seed
1 teaspoon mustard seed
3 packets sugar substitute

Yield: 12 ¼-cup servings or
3 cups relish

Food Exchange: Free

Combine jicama, cucumber, pimento, and salt in a
large mixing bowl. Let stand for 3 hours. Drain off
liquid. Combine vinegar, celery seed, mustard seed,
and sugar substitute in a saucepan. Bring to a boil.
Stir in vegetable mixture. Return to boiling. Boil
uncovered for 5 minutes. Pour into sterilized jars for
canning or refrigerate mixture in glass jars.

Calories per ¼ cup	15
Protein	0
Carbohydrate	4 g
Fat	0
Sodium	176 mg
Potassium	105 mg
Cholesterol	0

* A Central American root vegetable that looks like a large
brown turnip. Jicama has a crisp, slightly sweet taste and
can be found in any specialty greengrocer or market.

Curry Corn Relish

2 cups whole kernel corn
½ cup sliced, pitted ripe olives
¼ cup diced pimento
¼ cup olive oil
¼ cup cider vinegar
⅛ teaspoon ground white
   pepper
1 packet sugar substitute
½ teaspoon curry powder

Yield: 6 ⅓-cup servings

Food Exchanges: 1 starch/bread
+ 2 fats

Combine all ingredients in a large bowl. Mix thoroughly. Chill.

Calories per ⅓ cup	156
Protein	1 g
Carbohydrate	13 g
Fat	12 g
Sodium	232 mg
Potassium	67 mg
Cholesterol	0

Pickled Pears

3 cups low-calorie cranberry
   juice
½ cup wine vinegar
10 whole cloves
2 sticks cinnamon
2 teaspoons chopped
   crystallized ginger
1 teaspoon ground ginger
8 fresh ripe pears
8 packets sugar substitute

Yield: 16 servings of ½ pear or
3 pints

Food Exchange: 1 fruit

Combine cranberry juice, vinegar, cloves, cinnamon, and ginger in a large saucepan. Bring to a boil; reduce heat to simmer. Peel and core pears. Add to cranberry juice mixture. Simmer until pears are tender, about 10 minutes. Pack pears into hot, sterilized canning jars. Sprinkle sugar substitute over liquid and stir to dissolve. Pour liquid over pears. Seal jars using a hot water bath or store in the refrigerator until ready to use.

Calories per ½ pear	64
Protein	0
Carbohydrate	16 g
Fat	0
Sodium	1 mg
Potassium	117 mg
Cholesterol	0

Pickled Watermelon Rind

2 pounds watermelon rind
¼ cup salt
1 quart water
2 cups vinegar
2 cups water
2 sticks cinnamon
1 teaspoon whole cloves
1 teaspoon whole allspice
1 lemon, thinly sliced
8 packets sugar substitute

Peel watermelon rind and remove all pink. Cut into 2-inch-square cubes. Soak rind overnight in a brine made by dissolving the salt in 1 quart water. Drain and wash in fresh water. Cover rind with fresh water and cook until tender. Drain off water. Add vinegar, 2 cups water, cinnamon, cloves, allspice, and lemon. Cook until rind is clear. Remove from heat. Stir in sugar substitute. Pack into hot, sterilized jars. Cover with liquid and seal.

Calories per 6 cubes	37
Protein	0
Carbohydrate	8 g
Fat	0
Sodium	0
Potassium	102 mg
Cholesterol	0

Yield: 4 pints

Food Exchange: ½ fruit

Cheesy Snack Balls

1 cup chopped raisins
½ cup snipped apricots
½ cup chopped peanuts or
   sunflower seeds
1 cup grated American cheese
2 tablespoons peanut butter

Combine all ingredients in a bowl. Mix well with hands. Shape into balls. Chill.

Calories per 2 balls	65
Protein	2 g
Carbohydrate	7 g
Fat	4 g
Sodium	89 mg
Potassium	102 mg
Cholesterol	5 mg

Yield: 12 servings of 2 balls each

Food Exchanges: ½ starch/bread + 1 fat

Peanut Butter Popcorn

⅔ *cup unpopped popcorn*
1 *tablespoon margarine*
¼ *cup chunky peanut butter*

Pop popcorn in a hot-air popper. Melt margarine in a saucepan over low heat. Add peanut butter, stirring until melted. Drizzle peanut butter over popcorn. Toss lightly to mix.

Calories per cup	40
Protein	1 g
Carbohydrate	2 g
Fat	3 g
Sodium	33 mg
Potassium	25 mg
Cholesterol	0

Yield: 16 1-cup servings

Food Exchange: 1 fat

Herbed Popcorn

3 *cups popped popcorn*
½ *teaspoon dried oregano leaves*
½ *teaspoon ground coriander*
¼ *teaspoon ground cumin*

Combine all ingredients in a large bowl. Toss to mix.

Calories per 3 cups	85
Protein	3 g
Carbohydrate	17 g
Fat	1 g
Sodium	0
Potassium	73 mg
Cholesterol	0

Yield: 3 cups

Food Exchange: 1 starch/bread

8

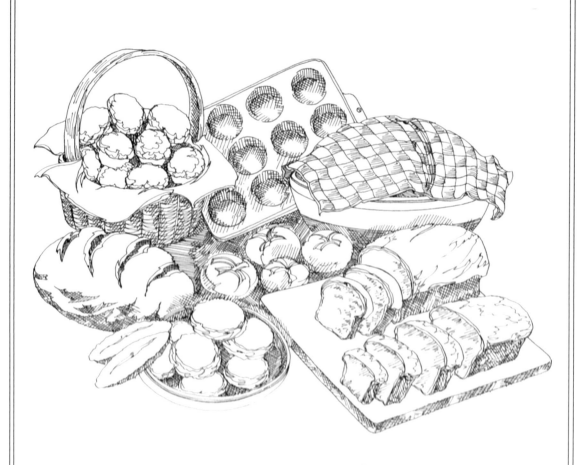

Breads

Oat Bran Muffins

3 egg whites
1 cup skim milk
2 tablespoons vegetable oil
2 cups oat bran
1 tablespoon baking powder
1 teaspoon ground cinnamon
2 tablespoons honey
¼ cup raisins
2 tablespoons chopped walnuts

Yield: 12 muffins

Food Exchanges: 1 starch/bread + 1 fat

Beat together egg whites, milk, and oil. Add oat bran, baking powder, cinnamon, honey, and raisins. Stir to mix. Fill lightly oiled or paper-lined muffin tins two-thirds full. Sprinkle walnuts on top. Bake in a 400-degree oven for 10 to 12 minutes.

Calories per muffin	108
Protein	4 g
Carbohydrate	15 g
Fats	4 g
Sodium	129 mg
Potassium	136 mg
Cholesterol	0

Oatmeal-Raisin Muffins

1¼ cups skim milk
3 tablespoons vegetable oil
1 cup rolled oats
1 egg
1 cup whole wheat flour
¼ cup sugar
½ cup raisins
1 tablespoon baking powder

Yield: 12 muffins

Food Exchanges: 1 starch/bread + 1 fat

Combine milk, oil, rolled oats, and egg in a bowl. Let stand for 5 minutes. Add remaining ingredients and stir until all ingredients are blended. Pour batter into lightly oiled muffin cups. Bake in a 400-degree oven for 10 to 12 minutes or until browned.

Calories per muffin	138
Protein	4 g
Carbohydrate	22 g
Fat	5 g
Sodium	104 mg
Potassium	161 mg
Cholesterol	23 mg

Oatmeal Muffins

1½ cups whole wheat flour
⅓ cup rolled oats
2 teaspoons baking powder
1 teaspoon sugar
1 egg
¾ cup skim milk
1 tablespoon vegetable oil

Yield: 8 muffins

Food Exchanges: 1 starch/bread + ½ fat

Combine flour, oats, baking powder, and sugar in mixing bowl. Stir to blend. Add egg, milk, and oil. Mix just until moistened. Spoon into oiled muffin cups. Bake in 375-degree oven for 10 to 15 minutes.

Calories per muffin	124
Protein	5 g
Carbohydrate	20 g
Fat	3 g
Sodium	95 mg
Potassium	147 mg
Cholesterol	35 mg

Variation: After mixing together all other ingredients, fold in ¼ cup chocolate chips.*

Calories per muffin	147
Protein	5 g
Carbohydrate	23 g
Fat	4 g
Sodium	96 mg
Potassium	147 mg
Cholesterol	35 mg

Food Exchanges: 1 starch/bread + 1 fat

* This recipe contains chocolate chips, which are high in saturated fat and sugar. Reserve this recipe variation for very special occasions only.

Mincemeat-Oatmeal Muffins

2½ cups whole wheat flour
1 cup rolled oats
1 tablespoon baking powder
1 teaspoon baking soda
1 cup mincemeat (see page 116)
1½ cups orange juice
3 tablespoons vegetable oil
1 egg
2 tablespoons honey

Yield: 18 muffins

Food Exchanges: 1 starch/bread
+ 1 fat

Combine all ingredients in a bowl. Mix just until blended. Pour into lightly oiled muffin cups. Bake in a 375-degree oven for 12 to 15 minutes.

Calories per muffin	156
Protein	4 g
Carbohydrate	24 g
Fat	4 g
Sodium	108 mg
Potassium	165 mg
Cholesterol	18 mg

Corn-Oatmeal Muffins

2 cups cornmeal
1 cup rolled oats
1 cup unbleached flour
2 tablespoons baking powder
1 teaspoon baking soda
2 tablespoons sugar
2 eggs
¼ cup vegetable oil
2 cups low-fat buttermilk (or
  sour milk)

Yield: 16 muffins

Food Exchanges: 1½ starches/
breads + 1 fat

Combine all ingredients in a mixing bowl. Stir just until mixed. Pour into lightly oiled muffin cups. Bake in a 375-degree oven for 15 to 20 minutes.

Calories per muffin	167
Protein	5 g
Carbohydrate	26 g
Fat	5 g
Sodium	201 mg
Potassium	106 mg
Cholesterol	35 mg

Vegetable-Corn Muffins

½ cup cornmeal
½ cup all-purpose flour
1 tablespoon sugar
1 tablespoon baking powder
⅛ teaspoon ground black
  pepper
1 tablespoon minced fresh dill
  weed or 1 teaspoon dried dill
  weed
1 egg
⅓ cup milk
1 tablespoon vegetable oil
¾ cup grated zucchini
¼ cup finely chopped red
  sweet pepper
¼ cup minced green onion

Combine all ingredients in a mixing bowl. Mix only until all ingredients are blended. Fill lightly oiled muffin cups three quarters of the way full. Bake in a 400-degree oven for 15 to 20 minutes, or until golden brown.

Calories per muffin	96
Protein	3 g
Carbohydrate	15 g
Fat	3 g
Sodium	107 mg
Potassium	72 mg
Cholesterol	34 mg

Yield: 8 muffins

Food Exchanges: 1 starch/bread
+ ½ fat

Corn Meal–Whole Wheat Muffins

1½ cups whole wheat flour
1 cup cornmeal
4 teaspoons baking powder
¼ cup sugar
1 egg
½ cup vegetable oil
1 cup skim milk

Combine flour, cornmeal, baking powder, and sugar in a mixing bowl. Add egg, oil, and milk. Stir just until moistened. Spoon into lightly oiled muffin cups. Bake in a 400-degree oven for 12 to 15 minutes.

Yield: 12 muffins

Food Exchanges: 1 starch/bread
+ 2 fats

Calories per muffin	187
Protein	4 g
Carbohydrate	21 g
Fat	10 g
Sodium	99 mg
Potassium	110 mg
Cholesterol	23 mg

Bran Cereal Muffins

¾ cup high-fiber bran cereal
1 cup skim milk
¾ cup all-purpose flour
2 teaspoons baking powder
2 tablespoons sugar
1 egg
2 tablespoons vegetable oil

Yield: 9 muffins

Food Exchanges: 1 starch/bread
+ 1 fat

Combine cereal and milk. Let stand for 5 minutes. Add remaining ingredients and mix just until all ingredients are blended. Spoon batter into lightly oiled muffin cups. Bake in a 400-degree oven for 15 to 20 minutes.

Calories per muffin	107
Protein	3 g
Carbohydrate	16 g
Fat	4 g
Sodium	148 mg
Potassium	140 mg
Cholesterol	31 mg

Pumpkin-Bran Muffins

1½ cups whole wheat flour
⅔ cup bran
1 tablespoon baking powder
½ teaspoon baking soda
1 teaspoon ground cinnamon
½ teaspoon ground nutmeg
¼ teaspoon ground cloves
1 cup pumpkin
1 egg
1 tablespoon honey
3 tablespoons oil
1 cup orange juice

Yield: 15 muffins

Food Exchanges: 1 starch/bread
+ ½ fat

Combine flour, bran, baking powder, baking soda, cinnamon, nutmeg, and cloves in a mixing bowl. Beat pumpkin, egg, honey, oil, and orange juice together. Add pumpkin mixture to flour mixture and mix just until ingredients are blended. Pour batter into lightly oiled muffin cups. Bake in a 400-degree oven for 12 to 15 minutes.

Calories per muffin	96
Protein	3 g
Carbohydrate	16 g
Fat	3 g
Sodium	98 mg
Potassium	165 mg
Cholesterol	18 mg

Carob-Bran Muffins

½ *cup wheat bran*
1 *cup whole wheat flour*
⅓ *cup carob powder*
2 *teaspoons baking powder*
½ *teaspoon baking soda*
½ *teaspoon ground cinnamon*
⅔ *cup skim milk*
2 *tablespoons vegetable oil*
1 *egg*

Yield: 8 muffins

Food Exchanges: 1 starch/bread
+ 1 fat

Combine bran, flour, carob powder, baking powder, baking soda, and cinnamon in a bowl. Add milk, oil, and egg. Stir just until all ingredients are moist. Spoon batter into lightly oiled muffin cups. Bake in a 400-degree oven for 12 to 15 minutes.

Calories per muffin	114
Protein	5 g
Carbohydrate	16 g
Fat	5 g
Sodium	133 mg
Potassium	186 mg
Cholesterol	35 mg

Italian Plum Muffins

½ *cup whole wheat flour*
½ *cup all-purpose flour*
1½ *teaspoons baking powder*
½ *teaspoon baking soda*
½ *teaspoon ground cinnamon*
¼ *teaspoon ground nutmeg*
2 *tablespoons vegetable oil*
1 *egg*
½ *cup skim milk*
2 *tablespoons honey*
⅔ *cup (about 4) chopped fresh*
  Italian prune plums

Yield: 6 muffins

Food Exchanges: 1 starch/bread
+ 1 fat

Combine all ingredients in a mixing bowl. Mix only until all ingredients are moistened. Spoon batter into lightly oiled muffin cups. Bake in a 350-degree oven for 15 to 20 minutes.

Calories per muffin	150
Protein	4 g
Carbohydrate	21 g
Fat	6 g
Sodium	153 mg
Potassium	96 mg
Cholesterol	46 mg

Cranberry Muffins

2 tablespoons vegetable oil
1 egg
⅓ cup skim milk
1 tablespoon honey
½ cup fresh or frozen
   cranberries, chopped
½ cup whole wheat flour
½ cup all-purpose flour
2 teaspoons baking powder
½ teaspoon ground cinnamon
½ cup chopped walnuts

Combine all ingredients in a mixing bowl. Stir just until moistened. Spoon batter into lightly oiled muffin cups. Bake in a 350-degree oven for 15 to 20 minutes.

Calories per muffin	207
Protein	5 g
Carbohydrate	21 g
Fat	12 g
Sodium	102 mg
Potassium	136 mg
Cholesterol	46 mg

Yield: 6 muffins

Food Exchanges: 1½ starches/ breads + 2 fats

Pear Muffins

1 pear
½ cup skim milk
2 tablespoons vegetable oil
1 egg
1 cup whole wheat flour
½ cup rolled oats
1 tablespoon sugar
½ teaspoon ground cinnamon
¼ cup raisins
2 teaspoons baking powder
½ teaspoon baking soda

Chop pear. Combine all ingredients in a mixing bowl. Stir just until blended. Spoon batter into lightly oiled muffin cups. Bake in a 400-degree oven for 15 to 20 minutes.

Calories per muffin	132
Protein	4 g
Carbohydrate	21 g
Fat	4 g
Sodium	131 mg
Potassium	132 mg
Cholesterol	31 mg

Yield: 9 muffins

Food Exchanges: 1 starch/bread + 1 fat

Carrot-Coconut Muffins

⅓ cup vegetable oil
½ cup sugar
1 egg
1¼ cups whole wheat flour
¼ teaspoon salt
2 teaspoons baking powder
½ teaspoon baking soda
½ teaspoon ground cinnamon
1 cup grated carrots
⅓ cup shredded coconut
⅓ cup skim milk

Yield: 10 muffins

Food Exchanges: 1 starch/bread + 2 fats

Beat together oil, sugar, and egg. Stir in remaining ingredients. Spoon into lightly oiled muffin cups. Bake in a 350-degree oven for 15 to 20 minutes.

Calories per muffin	180
Protein	3 g
Carbohydrate	23 g
Fat	9 g
Sodium	158 mg
Potassium	142 mg
Cholesterol	28 mg

Note: This recipe contains a moderate amount of sucrose. This recipe is for occasional use only and should be carefully worked into the individual meal plan.

Carrot-Coconut Passover Muffins

1 cup matzo meal
½ cup water
2 ripe bananas, mashed
1 carrot, grated
½ cup shredded coconut
1 apple, grated

Yield: 8 muffins

Food Exchanges: 1 starch/bread + ½ fruit

Combine all ingredients in a mixing bowl. Stir to blend. Spoon batter into 6 muffin cups. Bake in a 375-degree oven for 30 to 40 minutes, or until browned.

Calories per muffin	114
Protein	2 g
Carbohydrate	23 g
Fat	2 g
Sodium	6 g
Potassium	208 mg
Cholesterol	0

Herbed Popovers

1 cup all-purpose flour
¼ teaspoon salt
1 tablespoon minced green
    onion
¼ teaspoon dried marjoram
    leaves
¼ teaspoon dried thyme leaves
1 cup skim milk
2 eggs
2 tablespoons vegetable oil

Yield: 9 popovers

Food Exchanges: 1 starch/bread
+ 1 fat

Combine flour, salt, green onion, marjoram, and thyme in a bowl. Stir to blend. Add remaining ingredients and beat with a rotary beater until smooth. Pour batter into well-oiled, preheated popover pans or muffin cups. Bake in a 400-degree oven for 35 to 40 minutes, or until brown and crisp.

Calories per popover	101
Protein	4 g
Carbohydrate	11 g
Fat	4 g
Sodium	84 mg
Potassium	73 mg
Cholesterol	61 mg

Passover Popovers

1 cup water
½ cup vegetable oil
1 cup matzo meal
¼ teaspoon salt
2 tablespoons sugar
4 eggs

Yield: 12 popovers

Food Exchanges: 1 starch/bread
+ 2 fats

Combine water and oil in a saucepan. Bring to a boil; remove from heat. Add matzo meal, salt, and sugar. Mix well. Beat in 1 egg at a time. Fill oiled popover pans or muffin cups two-thirds full. Bake in a preheated 400-degree oven for 10 minutes. Reduce heat to 375 degrees and bake for 35 to 40 minutes longer, or until popovers are "popped."

Calories per popover	149
Protein	3 g
Carbohydrate	10 g
Fat	11 g
Sodium	64 mg
Potassium	31 mg
Cholesterol	91 mg

Oatmeal-Pumpkin Bread

¼ *cup vegetable oil*
3 *tablespoons sugar*
1 *egg*
1 *cup canned pumpkin*
1 *cup all-purpose flour*
½ *cup whole wheat flour*
2 *teaspoons baking powder*
½ *teaspoon baking soda*
1 *teaspoon ground cinnamon*
½ *teaspoon ground nutmeg*
¼ *teaspoon ground cloves*
½ *cup rolled oats*
½ *cup skim milk*
½ *cup chopped dates*

Beat together oil, sugar, egg, and pumpkin. Add remaining ingredients. Mix well to blend. Pour batter into an oiled loaf pan. Bake in a 350-degree oven for 50 to 55 minutes. Cool for 5 minutes in the pan before removing. Cool thoroughly before slicing.

Calories per slice	93
Protein	2 g
Carbohydrate	13 g
Fat	4 g
Sodium	22 mg
Potassium	86 mg
Cholesterol	15 mg

Yield: 1 loaf or 18 ½-inch slices

Food Exchange: 1 starch/bread

Carob-Raisin Bread

1 cup raisins

1 cup hot water (120 to 130
  degrees)

¼ cup sugar

¼ cup margarine

1 teaspoon grated orange peel

1 egg

2 cups whole wheat flour

1 tablespoon baking powder

½ teaspoon baking soda

⅓ cup carob powder

½ cup orange juice

½ cup chopped walnuts

Yield: 1 loaf or 15 1-inch slices

Food Exchanges: 1 starch/bread
+ ½ fruit + 1 fat

Combine raisins and water. Let stand for 10 minutes. Cream together sugar, margarine, orange peel, and egg. Add flour, baking powder, baking soda, carob powder, and orange juice. Stir in raisin mixture and walnuts. Mix just until all ingredients are moistened. Pour into a lightly oiled 9-by-5-by-3-inch baking pan. Bake in a 350-degree oven about 40 minutes. Cool for 5 minutes in the pan. Remove from the pan and cool thoroughly before slicing.

Calories per slice	162
Protein	4 g
Carbohydrate	25 g
Fat	7 g
Sodium	119 mg
Potassium	201 mg
Cholesterol	18 mg

Zucchini Bread

2 cups all-purpose flour
1 tablespoon baking powder
½ teaspoon ground cinnamon
¼ teaspoon ground nutmeg
2 tablespoons sugar
1 egg
⅓ cup vegetable oil
2 cups grated zucchini squash
½ cup orange juice or water

Yield: 1 loaf or 15 ½-inch slices

Food Exchanges: 1 starch/bread + 1 fat

Combine flour, baking powder, cinnamon, nutmeg, and sugar in a bowl. Beat egg, oil, and zucchini together. Add mixture to flour along with orange juice or water. Mix well. Pour batter into an oiled 9-by-5-inch loaf pan. Bake in a 350-degree oven for 40 to 45 minutes. Cool on a wire rack for 5 minutes before removing from pan. Cool thoroughly before slicing.

Calories per slice	116
Protein	2 g
Carbohydrate	15 g
Fat	5 g
Sodium	54 mg
Potassium	52 mg
Cholesterol	18 mg

Mincemeat-Banana Bread

2 cups whole wheat flour
2 teaspoons baking powder
1 teaspoon baking soda
1 egg
¼ cup vegetable oil
1 cup mincemeat (see page 116)
1 large ripe banana, mashed
½ cup apple juice

Yield: 1 loaf or 15 ½-inch slices

Food Exchanges: 1 starch/bread + 1 fat

Combine flour, baking powder, and baking soda. Stir to blend. Beat egg, oil, mincemeat, and banana together in another bowl. Combine mixtures. Add apple juice and mix well. Spoon into an oiled 9-by-5-inch loaf pan. Bake in a 350-degree oven for 40 to 50 minutes. Cool for 10 minutes before removing from pan. Cool thoroughly before slicing.

Calories per slice	145
Protein	3 g
Carbohydrate	22 g
Fat	5 g
Sodium	96 mg
Potassium	180 mg
Cholesterol	21 mg

Rhubarb-Nut Bread

½ cup sugar
½ cup vegetable oil
1 egg
½ cup orange juice
1⅓ cups whole wheat flour
2 teaspoons baking powder
½ teaspoon baking soda
1½ cups finely chopped
   rhubarb
¼ cup chopped walnuts

Beat together sugar, oil, egg, and juice. Add rest of the ingredients. Stir to blend well. Pour into oiled bread pan. Bake in 325-degree oven for 45 to 55 minutes, or until brown.

Calories per slice	186
Protein	3 g
Carbohydrate	20 g
Fat	11 g
Sodium	82 mg
Potassium	126 mg
Cholesterol	23 mg

Yield: 1 loaf or 12 1-inch slices

Food Exchanges: 1 starch/bread + 2 fats

Note: This recipe contains a moderate amount of sucrose. This recipe is for occasional use only and should be carefully worked into the individual meal plan.

Irish Soda Bread

2 cups all-purpose flour
2 teaspoons baking powder
½ teaspoon baking soda
¼ teaspoon salt
1 tablespoon caraway seeds
2 tablespoons sugar
½ cup raisins
½ cup buttermilk
2 eggs
⅓ cup margarine

Mix together flour, baking powder, baking soda, salt, caraway seeds, sugar, and raisins. Combine buttermilk, eggs, and margarine. Stir into flour mixture. Spoon into a lightly oiled springform pan or a 9-inch square baking pan. Bake in a 350-degree oven for 30 to 40 minutes or until crust is browned. Cool and remove from pan.

Calories per serving	117
Protein	3 g
Carbohydrate	17 g
Fat	5 g
Sodium	146 mg
Potassium	70 mg
Cholesterol	35 mg

Yield: 16 servings

Food Exchanges: 1 starch/bread + 1 fat

Sourdough Rye Bread

Starter Mixture

1 tablespoon dry yeast
2 cups warm water (110 degrees)
2 cups whole wheat flour
2 teaspoons sugar

Bread

2 cups rye flour
1 cup warm water (110 degrees)
1 tablespoon dry yeast
1 teaspoon salt
2 tablespoons caraway seeds
2 tablespoons sugar
1 tablespoon vegetable oil
2½ to 3 cups whole wheat flour
Cornmeal

To make starter mixture, dissolve 1 tablespoon dry yeast in 2 cups warm water. Add 2 cups whole wheat flour and 2 teaspoons sugar. Blend well. Batter will be lumpy. Cover and let stand in a warm place (70 to 80 degrees) for 3 days. Batter will separate, so stir it once or twice daily.

On the fourth day, combine 1 cup starter mixture with 2 cups rye flour. Add 1 cup warm water. Beat well. Cover and set in a warm place overnight. Replenish starter mixture by adding 1 cup whole wheat flour and 1 cup warm water to the remaining cup of starter mixture. Mix; cover and let stand overnight in a warm place. Pour starter mixture into a jar and refrigerate until needed. Use within 10 to 14 days.

On the fifth day, stir the rye batter. Add dry yeast, salt, caraway seeds, sugar, oil, and enough whole wheat flour to make a stiff dough.

Place dough onto a floured board. Knead dough at least 5 minutes. Place in an oiled bowl. Let rise in a warm place about 2 hours. Punch down and place on a floured board. Divide dough in half. Shape into 2 round loaves. Place on a lightly oiled baking sheet sprinkled with cornmeal. Make 2 or 3 slashes on top of each loaf. Cover with a towel and let rise in a warm place for 1 hour. Bake in a 400-degree oven for 30 to 35 minutes.

Yield: 2 loaves or 24 ½-inch slices

Food Exchange: 1 starch/bread

Calories per slice	102
Protein	4 g
Carbohydrate	21 g
Fat	1 g
Sodium	82 mg
Potassium	92 mg
Cholesterol	0

Italian Bread

1 tablespoon dry yeast
1 teaspoon sugar
⅔ cup warm water (110
  degrees)
2 tablespoons vegetable oil
½ teaspoon salt
2 cups all-purpose flour
Cornmeal
Egg white, slightly beaten

Dissolve yeast and sugar in water. Let stand for 5 minutes. Add oil, salt, and flour. Beat until dough is soft and well blended. Turn dough onto a lightly floured board. Knead and fold dough gently to mix in flour. Let dough rest for 5 minutes. Roll dough into a 12-by-6-inch rectangle. Form a loaf by rolling dough from the wide end. Oil a baking sheet. Sprinkle the sheet with cornmeal. Place loaf on the sheet. Let stand in a warm place until doubled in bulk, about 1 hour. Brush with egg white. Sprinkle top with cornmeal. Bake in a 425-degree oven for 35 to 40 minutes, or until loaf sounds hollow when tapped on crust. Cool.

Yield: 1 loaf or 15 1-inch slices

Food Exchange: 1 starch/bread

Calories per slice	74
Protein	2 g
Carbohydrate	12 g
Fat	2 g
Sodium	66 mg
Potassium	25 mg
Cholesterol	0

Strawberry Bread

1 cup all-purpose flour
½ cup whole wheat flour
1 teaspoon baking powder
½ teaspoon baking soda
¼ cup sugar
1 egg
⅓ cup vegetable oil
¾ cup orange juice or water
1½ cups sliced fresh
   strawberries
⅓ cup toasted sunflower seeds

Yield: 1 loaf or 15 1-inch slices

Food Exchanges: 1 starch/bread
+ 1 fat

Combine flours, baking powder, baking soda, and sugar in a mixing bowl. Stir to blend. Add egg, oil, and orange juice. Mix until all ingredients are blended. Fold in strawberries and sunflower seeds. Pour batter into an oiled and floured 8 ½-by-4 ½-inch loaf pan. Bake in a 350-degree oven for 50 to 55 minutes. Let cool for 10 minutes before removing from the pan. Turn out of the pan and cool before cutting.

Calories per slice	128
Protein	3 g
Carbohydrate	15 g
Fat	7 g
Sodium	50 mg
Potassium	103 mg
Cholesterol	18 mg

Pear-Nut Bread

1 large ripe pear, cored and
  chopped
1 egg
½ cup rolled oats
½ cup bran (flakes) cereal
3 tablespoons vegetable oil
2 tablespoons grated orange
  peel
1¼ cups whole wheat flour
2 tablespoons sugar
2 teaspoons baking powder
½ teaspoon baking soda
½ teaspoon ground cinnamon
½ cup chopped pecans

Yield: 1 loaf or 15 1-inch slices

Food Exchanges: 1 starch/bread
+ 1 fat

Combine pear, egg, rolled oats, bran cereal, oil, and orange peel in a bowl. Let stand for 10 minutes. In another mixing bowl, combine remaining ingredients. Stir to blend. Add pear mixture and beat until well blended. Pour into a lightly oiled loaf pan. Bake in a 350-degree oven for 50 to 60 minutes. Cool for 5 minutes on a wire rack before removing from the pan. Cool thoroughly before slicing.

Calories per slice	117
Protein	3 g
Carbohydrate	14 g
Fat	6 g
Sodium	86 mg
Potassium	92 mg
Cholesterol	18 mg

50-Percent Whole Wheat Bread

½ cup water
¼ cup honey
1 teaspoon salt
⅓ cup vegetable oil
¾ cup skim milk
1 cup wheat bran
2 tablespoons dry yeast
¾ cup warm water (110
   degrees)
3 cups whole wheat flour
2 to 2¼ cups all-purpose flour

Combine ½ cup water, honey, salt, oil, milk, and bran in a large mixing bowl. Dissolve yeast in ¾ cup warm water. Combine mixtures and add whole wheat flour. Beat until smooth. Stir in enough all-purpose flour to make a stiff dough. Turn dough onto a floured surface and knead until smooth and elastic. Place in an oiled bowl; cover with a damp cloth and let rise in a warm place until doubled in bulk, about 1 hour. Punch down. Shape into a loaf on a floured surface. Place in a lightly oiled baking pan. Cover and let rise until doubled in bulk, about 30 minutes. Bake in a 400-degree oven for 50 minutes, or until loaf sounds hollow when tapped with a spoon. Cool before slicing.

Yield: 2 loaves or 30 ½-inch slices

Food Exchanges: 1 starch/bread + ½ fat

Calories per slice	105
Protein	3 g
Carbohydrate	18 g
Fat	3 g
Sodium	69 mg
Potassium	93 mg
Cholesterol	0

Oatmeal Bread

1 cup rolled oats
1 cup boiling water
2 tablespoons dry yeast
2 tablespoons sugar +
1 teaspoon sugar
½ cup warm water (110
   degrees)
1 cup skim milk
1 teaspoon salt
2½ cups whole wheat flour
2 to 2½ cups all-purpose flour

Place rolled oats in a mixing bowl. Pour boiling water over oats and stir to blend. Let stand for 5 minutes to thicken. Combine yeast, sugar, and ½ cup warm water in a bowl. Allow to stand until bubbly, about 5 minutes. Add yeast mixture, milk, salt, and whole wheat flour to oatmeal. Beat well. Add enough all-purpose flour to make a stiff dough, using ½ cup at a time. Turn dough out onto a floured board. Knead until smooth and elastic, adding extra flour as needed (about 5 minutes). Shape dough into a ball and place in an oiled bowl. Cover with a damp towel and let rise until doubled in bulk, about 1 hour. Punch down. Knead for 1 minute and shape into a loaf. Place into an oiled 8-by-4-inch baking pan. Cover and let rise until doubled in bulk. Bake in a 375-degree oven for 50 to 55 minutes, or until loaf is browned and sounds hollow when tapped with a spoon. Remove loaf from the pan. Cool thoroughly before slicing.

Yield: 1 loaf or 15 1-inch slices

Food Exchanges: 2 starches/breads

Calories per slice	158
Protein	6 g
Carbohydrate	32 g
Fat	1 g
Sodium	158 mg
Potassium	161 mg
Cholesterol	0

Cheese Pizza Bread

1 tablespoon dry yeast
1½ cups warm water (110 degrees)
1 tablespoon sugar
3 cups all-purpose flour
1 to 1½ cups whole wheat flour
1 teaspoon salt
3 tablespoons vegetable oil
½ cup shredded low-fat mozzarella cheese
1 teaspoon dried oregano leaves
½ teaspoon dried thyme leaves
⅛ teaspoon ground pepper

Yield: 1 loaf or 12 1-inch slices

Food Exchanges: 2 starches/ breads + ½ fat

Dissolve yeast in warm water. Add sugar. Beat in 3 cups all-purpose flour, 1 cup whole wheat flour, salt, oil, and cheese. Stir until well blended. Turn onto a lightly floured board. Knead for 5 to 7 minutes, or until smooth and elastic. Set to rise in an oiled bowl. Cover with a towel for about 1 hour. Punch down when doubled in bulk. Roll out into an 11-by-6-inch rectangle. Roll up into a loaf. Place in an oiled loaf pan. Sprinkle on oregano, thyme, and pepper. Let rise in a warm place until doubled in bulk. Bake in a 375-degree oven for 25 to 30 minutes. Cool and remove from pan.

Calories per slice	187
Protein	6 g
Carbohydrate	30 g
Fat	5 g
Sodium	186 mg
Potassium	82 mg
Cholesterol	3 mg

Feta Cheese Casserole Bread

1 tablespoon dry yeast

¼ cup warm water (110 degrees)

1 cup crumbled feta cheese, room temperature

½ cup plain low-fat yogurt, room temperature

1 egg

2 tablespoons honey

1 tablespoon margarine, softened

1 tablespoon dill seeds

3 to 3¼ cups whole wheat flour

2 tablespoons finely chopped onions

Yield: 1 loaf or 15 1-inch slices

Food Exchanges: 1 starch/bread + 1 fat

Soften yeast in warm water. Stir to dissolve. Add feta cheese, yogurt, egg, honey, margarine, dill seeds, and 2 cups flour. Beat well. Add onions and enough additional flour to make a stiff dough. Place in an oiled bowl and let rise in a warm place about 1 hour, or until doubled in bulk. Punch down. Knead for 30 seconds in the bowl. Place dough in an oiled casserole. Let rise in a warm place until doubled in bulk, about 30 minutes. Bake in a 350-degree oven about 30 minutes. Cool for 5 minutes in the casserole before serving.

Calories per slice	127
Protein	5 g
Carbohydrate	20 g
Fat	3 g
Sodium	104 mg
Potassium	130 mg
Cholesterol	25 mg

Basil and Cheese Bread Sticks

1 tablespoon dry yeast
1 teaspoon sugar
1 ½ cups warm water (110 degrees)
½ teaspoon salt
½ teaspoon ground black pepper
2 tablespoons dried basil leaves
1 tablespoon vegetable oil
½ cup grated Parmesan or Romano cheese
5 cloves garlic, minced
4 dashes Tabasco sauce
2 cups whole wheat flour
2 cups all-purpose flour

Yield: 20 bread sticks

Food Exchange: 1 starch/bread

Dissolve yeast and sugar in warm water. Let stand for 5 minutes. Add remaining ingredients, reserving ½ cup flour for kneading. Beat well. Turn onto a lightly floured surface and knead about 5 minutes until smooth. Add extra all-purpose flour as needed. Divide dough in half. Roll each half ½ inch thick. Cut into 10 strips. Roll and twist each strip into a rounded stick 12 inches long. Place on a lightly oiled baking sheet. Cover and let rise in a warm place about 30 minutes. Bake in a 350-degree oven for 15 to 20 minutes, or until lightly browned.

Calories per bread stick	101
Protein	4 g
Carbohydrate	18 g
Fat	2 g
Sodium	87 mg
Potassium	69 mg
Cholesterol	2 mg

Old-Fashioned Corn Sticks

2 cups cornmeal
3 teaspoons baking powder
1 tablespoon honey
1 egg
2 tablespoons vegetable oil
½ cup creamed or canned corn
1½ cups skim milk

Yield: 16 corn sticks

Food Exchanges: 1 starch/bread + 1 fat

Combine all ingredients in a mixing bowl and beat well. Pour into an oiled corn-stick pan or an 8-inch square baking pan. Bake in a 400-degree oven for 18 to 20 minutes.

Calories per corn stick	125
Protein	3 g
Carbohydrate	19 g
Fat	4 g
Sodium	24 mg
Potassium	74 mg
Cholesterol	18 mg

Bran Buttermilk Biscuits

1 cup whole wheat flour
¼ cup wheat bran*
¼ teaspoon baking soda
2 teaspoons baking powder
3 tablespoons margarine
⅓ cup buttermilk or ⅓ cup
   skim milk plus 1 teaspoon
   vinegar

Combine flour, bran, baking soda, and baking powder in a mixing bowl. Cut in margarine with a pastry blender or a knife. Add milk. Beat until smooth. Pat dough onto a floured surface until ½ inch thick. Cut into biscuits. Bake in a 400-degree oven for 10 to 12 minutes.

Calories per biscuit	97
Protein	3 g
Carbohydrate	12 g
Fat	5 g
Sodium	148 mg
Potassium	92 mg
Cholesterol	0

Yield: 8 biscuits

Food Exchanges: 1 starch/bread + 1 fat

* ½ cup 100-percent bran cereal can be substituted for ¼ cup wheat bran. Increase milk to ⅔ cup.

Zucchini Spoonbread

1 large zucchini (about 1
pound)
1 cup skim milk
1 tablespoon margarine
1 cup cornmeal
½ teaspoon baking powder
1 teaspoon dried marjoram
leaves
½ cup grated low-fat Gouda
cheese
4 eggs, separated

Yield: 6 servings

Food Exchanges: 1 medium-fat
meat + 1 starch/bread + 1 vegetable

Shred zucchini in a food processor. Combine milk
and margarine in a saucepan over medium heat.
Cook to melt margarine. Stir in cornmeal. Remove
from heat. Add zucchini, baking powder, marjoram,
cheese, and egg yolks. Mix well. Beat egg whites
until stiff. Fold egg whites into zucchini mixture.
Pour into a lightly oiled casserole. Bake in a 350-
degree oven for 40 to 45 minutes. Serve immediately.

Calories per serving	199
Protein	10 g
Carbohydrate	22 g
Fat	8 g
Sodium	154 mg
Potassium	196 mg
Cholesterol	189 mg

Note: This recipe contains more than ½ egg per serving.

Kulich

4½ cups all-purpose flour
¼ cup sugar
2 packages dry active yeast
½ teaspoon salt
1 teaspoon ground nutmeg
½ cup skim milk
¼ cup water
¼ cup vegetable oil
2 eggs
1 teaspoon vanilla
½ cup chopped almonds
½ cup raisins
½ cup chopped dried fruit
   (apricots, dates, peaches)

Combine 3½ cups flour, sugar, yeast, salt, and nutmeg in a large mixing bowl. Heat milk, water, and oil in a small saucepan just until lukewarm. Add to flour mixture with eggs and vanilla. Beat well. Stir in enough extra flour to make a soft dough. Add almonds, raisins, and fruit. Knead on a lightly floured board for 4 minutes, or until dough is smooth.

Place dough in a well-greased 2-pound coffee can or 2 46-ounce fruit juice cans. Cover with plastic wrap. Let rise in a warm place until doubled in bulk, about 20 minutes. Remove plastic wrap and bake in a 350-degree oven for 30 to 35 minutes. Tap the can gently on the sides to loosen. Remove from the can and cool on a wire rack.

Yield: 20 1-inch slices

Food Exchanges: 1 starch/bread + 1 fruit + 1 fat

Calories per slice	167
Protein	5 g
Carbohydrate	27 g
Fat	5 g
Sodium	60 mg
Potassium	124 mg
Cholesterol	28 mg

Mincemeat Swirls

1 tablespoon dry yeast
¼ cup warm water (110 degrees)
⅓ cup skim milk
2 tablespoons sugar
¼ cup margarine
½ teaspoon salt
1 egg
2 to 2¼ cups whole wheat flour
1 cup mincemeat (see page 116)

Dissolve yeast in warm water. Heat milk, sugar, and margarine in a saucepan until margarine melts. Cool. Add yeast mixture, salt, egg, and 2 cups flour. Beat until smooth. Add extra flour, if needed, to make a stiff batter. Refrigerate for 2 hours or overnight. Place dough on a lightly floured surface and roll into a 12-by-9-inch rectangle. Spread with mincemeat. Roll up jelly-roll fashion, starting with the long side. Seal edges. Cut into 12 slices. Place each in an oiled muffin cup with cut side up. Cover and let rise in a warm place about 1 hour, or until doubled in bulk. Bake in a 350-degree oven for 20 to 25 minutes, or until golden brown. Serve warm.

Yield: 12 buns

Food Exchanges: 1 starch/bread + ½ fruit + 1 fat

Calories per bun	163
Protein	5 g
Carbohydrate	24 g
Fat	5 g
Sodium	139 mg
Potassium	163 mg
Cholesterol	26 mg

Greek Christmas Loaf

1 tablespoon dry yeast

1 tablespoon sugar

½ cup warm water (110 degrees)

3 cups all-purpose flour

2 tablespoons margarine, soft

⅓ cup sugar

2 eggs

½ cup dried figs

2 teaspoons anise seeds

⅓ cup walnuts

2½ teaspoons grated orange peel

½ teaspoon anise extract

¼ cup golden raisins

Dissolve yeast and 1 tablespoon sugar in warm water in a food processor with a steel blade. Process mixture twice in on-off pulses. Let stand until yeast is foamy, about 5 minutes. Add flour, margarine, ⅓ cup sugar, and eggs. Process until dough sticks together and is smooth. Place dough in an oiled bowl. Turn dough to coat all sides with oil. Cover with a damp towel and let rise in a warm place until doubled in bulk, about 30 minutes. Prepare filling by combining remaining ingredients in a food processor with a steel blade. Process with on-off pulses until evenly chopped. When dough has doubled, punch down. Turn onto a lightly floured surface and knead for 1 minute. Roll on a lightly floured surface into a 12-by-4-inch rectangle. Spread filling on dough. Roll up dough, starting with the long side. Twist dough to coil. Cover loaf and let rise in a warm place until doubled, about 30 minutes. Bake in a 400-degree oven for 25 to 30 minutes, or until browned.

Yield: 1 loaf or 18 1-inch slices

Food Exchange: 1 starch/bread

Calories per slice	102
Protein	3 g
Carbohydrate	19 g
Fat	2 g
Sodium	9 mg
Potassium	83 mg
Cholesterol	30 mg

Cardamom Christmas Ring

2 cups whole wheat flour
1 teaspoon ground cardamom
1 tablespoon dry yeast
1 cup milk
⅓ cup vegetable oil
¼ cup sugar
½ teaspoon salt
2 eggs, separated
2 to 2½ cups all-purpose flour
2 tablespoons sugar
1 cup chopped pecans
1 cup snipped dried apricots
1 cup raisins or currants
Confectioner's sugar

Combine whole wheat flour, cardamom, and yeast in a bowl. Heat milk, oil, ¼ cup sugar, and salt just until warm (110 degrees). Add to flour mixture with egg yolks. Beat with an electric mixer for 3 minutes. Stir in enough all-purpose flour to make a stiff dough. Turn onto a lightly floured surface. Knead about 3 minutes to make a smooth elastic dough. Place in an oiled bowl and turn dough to coat all sides. Cover and let rise in a warm place until doubled in bulk (about 1 hour). Punch down. Divide in half. Let dough rest while combining egg whites, 2 tablespoons sugar, pecans, apricots, and raisins. Roll each half of dough on a floured surface into an 18-by-14-inch rectangle. Spread half of nut mixture on dough. Roll up. Shape into a ring by sealing edges. Place on an oiled baking sheet. Using a sharp knife or scissors, make 8 V-shaped cuts along the edge of the ring. Repeat with remaining dough. Cover and let rise until doubled in bulk (about 30 minutes). Bake in a 350-degree oven for 20 minutes or until browned. Cool. Sprinkle on confectioner's sugar just before serving.

Yield: 24 1-inch wedges

Food Exchanges: 1 starch/bread + ½ fruit + 1 fat

Calories per wedge	177
Protein	4 g
Carbohydrate	25 g
Fat	7 g
Sodium	53 mg
Potassium	191 mg
Cholesterol	23 mg

Hot Cross Buns

¼ *cup sugar*
½ *teaspoon salt*
½ *teaspoon ground cinnamon*
1 *package dry yeast*
4 *to 5 cups all-purpose flour*
½ *cup vegetable oil*
1 *cup skim milk*
1 *egg*
½ *cup raisins*
2 *teaspoons grated orange peel*
Sugar substitute

Combine sugar, salt, cinnamon, yeast, and 1 cup flour in a mixing bowl. Heat oil and milk in a small saucepan just until lukewarm. Add milk to flour mixture and beat with a mixer. Beat in egg and another cup of flour. Continue beating in extra flour with a wooden spoon to make a soft dough. Add raisins and orange peel. Turn dough onto a lightly floured board and knead until smooth and elastic. Shape into a ball. Place into an oiled bowl, turning to coat top of dough. Cover and let rise in a warm place until dough is doubled, about 1 hour.

Lightly oil a 9-by-13-inch baking pan. Punch dough down and divide into 18 pieces. Shape each piece into a ball. Arrange balls in the pan. Cover and let rise in a warm place until doubled, about 1 hour. Bake in a 375-degree oven for 20 to 25 minutes, or until golden brown. Remove buns from the pan; cool on a rack. Sprinkle sugar substitute on top.

Yield: 18 buns

Food Exchanges: 1 starch/bread + 1 fruit + 1 fat

Calories per bun	180
Protein	4 g
Carbohydrate	26 g
Fat	7 g
Sodium	69 mg
Potassium	92 mg
Cholesterol	15 mg

Zucchini Yeast Buns

2 to 2½ cups all-purpose flour
1 cup whole wheat flour
2 tablespoons sugar
1 tablespoon dry yeast
¼ cup water
¼ cup vegetable oil
2 small zucchini, sliced
1 egg

Combine 1 ½ cups all-purpose flour, whole wheat flour, sugar, and yeast in a mixing bowl. Stir to blend. In a blender or food processor, combine water, oil, and zucchini. Purée until smooth. Add zucchini and egg to flour mixture. Beat until smooth. Add extra flour to make a smooth soft dough. Cover and let rise in a warm place until doubled in bulk, about 1 hour. Punch down and divide into 18 balls. Place balls in two oiled 8-inch cake pans. Cover and let rise in a warm place until doubled, about 20 minutes. Bake in a 375-degree oven for 18 to 20 minutes, or until golden brown. Remove from pans and serve hot or cold.

Yield: 18 buns

Food Exchanges: 2 starches/breads + ½ fat

Calories per bun	108
Protein	3 g
Carbohydrate	16 g
Fat	4 g
Sodium	5 mg
Potassium	65 mg
Cholesterol	15 mg

Oatmeal Scones

1 cup unbleached flour
½ cup oatmeal
2 teaspoons baking powder
3 tablespoons margarine
½ cup skim milk
¼ cup raisins

Stir flour, oatmeal, and baking powder together in a bowl. Cut in margarine with a pastry blender or a fork. Add milk and mix into a soft dough. Pour dough onto a lightly floured surface. Sprinkle raisins on top. Knead dough to mix raisins and make a smooth dough. Roll or press out until ½ inch thick. Cut with a biscuit cutter or a glass. Place on a lightly oiled baking sheet. Bake in a 400-degree oven for 10 to 12 minutes.

Yield: 8 scones

Food Exchanges: 1 starch/bread + 1 fat

Calories per scone	128
Protein	3 g
Carbohydrate	19 g
Fat	5 g
Sodium	137 mg
Potassium	99 mg
Cholesterol	0

Oatmeal Waffles

1 egg
1 cup skim milk
2 tablespoons vegetable oil
½ cup rolled oats
1 cup whole wheat flour
1½ teaspoons baking powder
½ teaspoon baking soda
1 tablespoon sugar

Yield: 8 servings of ½ waffle or
4 4-inch waffles

Food Exchanges: 1 starch/bread
+ 1 fat

Beat egg, milk, and oil. Stir in rolled oats, flour, baking powder, baking soda, and sugar. Mix until smooth. Pour batter onto an oiled, preheated waffle iron. Cook until browned.

Calories per ½ waffle	125
Protein	5 g
Carbohydrate	17 g
Fat	5 g
Sodium	139 mg
Potassium	138 mg
Cholesterol	35 mg

Orange French Toast

1 egg
¼ cup skim milk
¼ teaspoon cinnamon
4 slices day-old whole wheat
    bread
1 tablespoon soft margarine
2 teaspoons grated orange peel
1 tablespoon orange juice
    concentrate
Sugar substitute

Yield: 4 slices

Food Exchanges: 1 starch/bread
+ 1 fat

Beat egg, milk, and cinnamon together with a fork. Brush a skillet lightly with oil and place over medium heat. Dip both sides of bread into egg mixture. Place in the skillet and brown well on each side. Place toast slices on a baking sheet. Blend margarine, orange peel, and concentrate together. Spread over bread slices. Just before serving, broil 3 inches from broiler until bubbly and brown. Sprinkle with sugar substitute before serving.

Calories per slice	118
Protein	5 g
Carbohydrate	15 g
Fat	5 g
Sodium	180 mg
Potassium	141 mg
Cholesterol	69 mg

Sourdough Coffeecake

1 cup sourdough starter (see page 137)
2 cups whole wheat flour
1 cup warm (110 degrees) water
1 tablespoon dry yeast
1 teaspoon salt
½ cup raisins
½ cup sugar
2 tablespoons vegetable oil
2½ to 3½ cups whole wheat flour
¼ cup margarine
⅓ cup brown sugar
½ cup chopped nuts

Combine starter, 2 cups whole wheat flour, and warm water. Beat well. Cover and set in a warm place overnight. The next day, add yeast, salt, raisins, sugar, oil, and enough whole wheat flour to make a stiff dough. Place dough in an oiled bowl and let rise in a warm place about 1 hour, or until doubled in bulk. Punch down and place on a lightly floured board or cloth. Flatten dough with a rolling pin and shape into a 24-by-12-inch rectangle. Spread margarine on top. Sprinkle on brown sugar and nuts. Roll up jelly-roll fashion. Cut into 24 1-inch pieces. Arrange in a lightly oiled tube pan. Let rise until doubled, about ½ hour. Bake in a 350-degree oven for 40 to 50 minutes.

Calories per slice	175
Protein	5 g
Carbohydrate	30 g
Fat	5 g
Sodium	106 mg
Potassium	149 mg
Cholesterol	0

Yield: 1 coffeecake or 24 1-inch slices

Food Exchanges: 1 starch/bread + 1 fruit + 1 fat

Note: This recipe contains a moderate amount of sucrose. This recipe is for occasional use only and should be carefully worked into the individual meal plan.

9

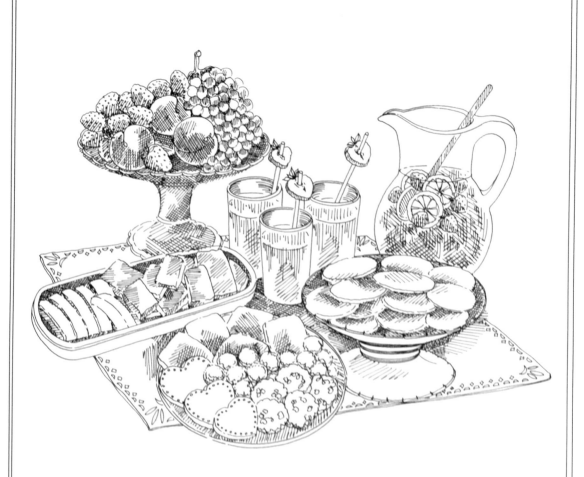

Cookies

Chocolate Chip Cookies

¾ *cup vegetable oil*

¼ *cup sugar*

¼ *cup brown sugar*

1 *egg*

1 *teaspoon vanilla extract*

1 *teaspoon baking powder*

½ *teaspoon baking soda*

1¾ *cups all-purpose flour*

½ *cup chocolate chips*

⅓ *cup chopped walnuts*

Cream together oil, sugars, egg, and vanilla. Add baking powder, baking soda, flour, chocolate chips,* and nuts. Stir to blend well.** Drop by spoonfuls onto a lightly oiled baking sheet. Bake in 375-degree oven 10 to 12 minutes.

Calories per 2 cookies	136
Protein	1 g
Carbohydrate	12 g
Fat	8 g
Sodium	32 mg
Potassium	24 mg
Cholesterol	12 mg

Yield: 48 cookies

Food Exchanges: 1 starch/bread + 1 fat

* This recipe contains chocolate chips, which are high in saturated fat and sugar. Reserve this recipe for very special occasions only.

** Two tablespoons of water may be added if batter does not stick together.

Hazelnut Cookies

¼ *cup margarine*

⅓ *cup sugar*

1 egg

½ *teaspoon vanilla extract*

½ *cup whole wheat flour*

½ *cup all-purpose flour*

2 teaspoons baking powder

½ *cup coarsely chopped*
hazelnuts

1 teaspoon grated orange peel

Yield: 36 cookies

Food Exchange: ½ starch/bread

Cream together margarine, sugar, egg, and vanilla. Add rest of ingredients and beat well. Drop by spoonfuls onto a lightly oiled baking sheet. Bake in 350-degree oven for 10 to 12 minutes or until golden brown.

Calories per cookie	40
Protein	1 g
Carbohydrate	4 g
Fat	2 g
Sodium	31 mg
Potassium	16 mg
Cholesterol	8 mg

Variation: After mixing together all other ingredients, fold in ½ cup chocolate chips.*

Calories per cookie	52
Protein	1 g
Carbohydrate	6 g
Fat	3 g
Sodium	31 mg
Potassium	16 mg
Cholesterol	8 mg

Food Exchanges: ½ starch/bread + ½ fat

* This recipe variation contains chocolate chips, which are high in saturated fat and sugar. Reserve this recipe variation for very special occasions only.

Pumpkin Cookies

⅓ cup vegetable oil
1 cup sugar
1 cup canned pumpkin
1 egg
1 teaspoon vanilla extract
2 cups whole wheat flour
1½ teaspoons baking powder
½ teaspoon baking soda
1 teaspoon ground cinnamon
¼ teaspoon ground nutmeg
½ cup chopped pecans

Yield: 36 cookies

Food Exchanges: 1 starch/bread + ½ fat

Cream together oil, sugar, pumpkin, egg, and vanilla. Add flour, baking powder, baking soda, cinnamon, and nutmeg. Stir to blend well. Add pecans. Drop by teaspoonfuls onto a lightly oiled baking sheet. Bake in 350-degree oven for 10 to 12 minutes.

Calories per cookie	76
Protein	1 g
Carbohydrate	11 g
Fat	3 g
Sodium	35 mg
Potassium	50 mg
Cholesterol	8 mg

Variation: Fold in 1 cup chocolate chips* when you add the pecans.

Calories per cookie	96
Protein	2 g
Carbohydrate	13 g
Fat	5 g
Sodium	36 mg
Potassium	50 mg
Cholesterol	8 mg

Food Exchanges: 1 starch/bread + 1 fat

* This recipe variation contains chocolate chips, which are high in saturated fat and sugar. Reserve this recipe variation for very special occasions only.

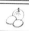
Trailside Oatmeal Treats

½ *cup vegetable oil*
½ *cup peanut butter*
1 *cup sugar*
2 *eggs*
½ *cup skim milk*
2 *cups whole wheat flour*
1 *teaspoon baking soda*
2 *cups rolled oats*
½ *cup raisins*
¼ *cup wheat germ, toasted*

Yield: 48 cookies

Food Exchanges: 1 starch/bread
+ 1 fat

Beat together oil, peanut butter, sugar, eggs, and milk. Add rest of ingredients and mix thoroughly. Drop by spoonfuls onto a lightly oiled baking sheet. Bake in 350-degree oven for about 10 minutes.

Calories per cookie	90
Protein	2 g
Carbohydrate	12 g
Fat	4 g
Sodium	48 mg
Potassium	72 mg
Cholesterol	11 mg

Variation: After mixing together all other ingredients, fold in ½ cup chocolate chips.*

Calories per cookie	98
Protein	2 g
Carbohydrate	13 g
Fat	5 g
Sodium	48 mg
Potassium	72 mg
Cholesterol	11 mg

Food Exchanges: 1 starch/bread
+ 1 fat

* This recipe variation contains chocolate chips, which are high in saturated fat and sugar. Reserve this recipe variation for very special occasions only.

Peanut Butter Oatmeal Munchies

⅓ cup vegetable oil
⅓ cup peanut butter
½ cup honey
2 eggs
¼ cup skim milk
1⅓ cups whole wheat flour
1 teaspoon baking powder
½ teaspoon baking soda
¾ cup rolled oats
½ cup raisins
¼ cup toasted sunflower seeds

Yield: 36 cookies

Food Exchanges: 1 starch/bread
+ 1 fat

Beat together oil, peanut butter, honey, eggs, and milk. Add rest of ingredients and mix until thoroughly blended. Drop by spoonfuls onto an ungreased baking sheet. Bake in 350-degree oven for about 10 minutes.

Calories per cookie	81
Protein	2 g
Carbohydrate	10 g
Fat	4 g
Sodium	50 mg
Potassium	69 mg
Cholesterol	15 mg

Variation: After mixing together all other ingredients, fold in ½ cup chocolate chips.*

Calories per cookie	95
Protein	2 g
Carbohydrate	12 g
Fat	5 g
Sodium	57 mg
Potassium	74 mg
Cholesterol	15 mg

* This recipe variation contains chocolate chips, which are high in saturated fat and sugar. Reserve this recipe variation for very special occasions only.

Food Exchanges: 1 starch/bread
+ 1 fat

Chocolate Date Balls

½ cup chopped pitted dates
40 vanilla wafers, finely
   crushed
2 tablespoons cocoa
4 tablespoons frozen orange
   juice concentrate

Yield: 36 cookies

Food Exchange: 1 starch/bread

Combine dates, vanilla wafers, cocoa, and orange juice concentrate. Mix well. Roll into small balls. Store in a tightly covered container.

Calories per 2 cookies	58
Protein	1 g
Carbohydrate	12 g
Fat	2 g
Sodium	22 mg
Potassium	66 mg
Cholesterol	0

Date Bars

¼ cup brown sugar
½ cup margarine
1 cup whole wheat flour
2 eggs
1 cup chopped pitted dates
½ cup chopped nuts
½ cup shredded coconut

Yield: 25 bars

Food Exchanges: ½ starch/bread
+ 1 fat

Cream sugar and margarine together until light and fluffy. Stir in flour. Press mixture into the bottom of an 8-inch square baking pan. Bake in a 350-degree oven for 10 minutes. Beat eggs, dates, nuts, and coconut. Spread over baked crust. Bake in a 350-degree oven for 20 minutes more or until top is golden. Cool before cutting.

Calories per bar	93
Protein	2 g
Carbohydrate	9 g
Fat	6 g
Sodium	49 mg
Potassium	69 mg
Cholesterol	22 mg

Orange-Date Bars

1 cup chopped dates
1/3 cup sugar
1/3 cup vegetable oil
1/2 cup orange juice
1 cup all-purpose flour
1/2 cup chopped pecans
1 egg
1 1/2 teaspoons baking powder
1 tablespoon grated orange
   rind

Yield: 36 bars

Food Exchanges: 1/2 starch/bread
+ 1/2 fat

Combine dates, sugar, oil, and juice in a saucepan. Cook for 5 minutes to soften dates. Cool. Add remaining ingredients. Spread into an oiled 8-inch baking pan. Bake in a 350-degree oven for 25 to 30 minutes. Cool before cutting.

Calories per bar	56
Protein	1 g
Carbohydrate	6 g
Fat	3 g
Sodium	12 mg
Potassium	34 mg
Cholesterol	8 mg

Black Walnut Squares

1/3 cup margarine
1/3 cup sugar
1 tablespoon grated orange
   peel
1 teaspoon vanilla extract
2 egg yolks
2/3 cup all-purpose flour
1 1/2 teaspoons baking powder
2/3 cup chopped black walnuts
2 egg whites

Yield: 35 squares

Food Exchanges: 1/2 starch/bread
+ 1 fat

Cream together margarine and sugar. Add orange peel, vanilla, and egg yolks. Beat until light and fluffy. Stir in flour and baking powder. Spread into a lightly oiled 9-inch square baking pan. Grind walnuts in a food processor or blender to coarse texture. Beat egg whites until stiff peaks. Fold in nuts. Spread nut mixture over cookie dough. Bake in a 375-degree oven for 25 to 30 minutes, or until brown.

Calories per 2 squares	96
Protein	2 g
Carbohydrate	8 g
Fat	6 g
Sodium	68 mg
Potassium	34 mg
Cholesterol	32 mg

Brownies

½ cup sugar
½ cup cocoa
⅓ cup vegetable oil
2 eggs
1 cup all-purpose flour
1 teaspoon baking powder
½ teaspoon baking soda
¼ cup chopped nuts

Yield: 32 brownies

Food Exchanges: ½ starch/bread + 1 fat

Beat together sugar, cocoa, oil, and eggs. Add remaining ingredients and stir until smooth. Bake in a lightly oiled 8-inch square pan for 25 to 30 minutes in a 350-degree oven.

Calories per brownie	59
Protein	1 g
Carbohydrate	7 g
Fat	4 g
Sodium	25 mg
Potassium	33 mg
Cholesterol	17 mg

Bran Brownies

½ cup vegetable oil
⅓ cup brown sugar
2 eggs
1 cup whole wheat flour
1 cup bran cereal
½ teaspoon baking soda
1 teaspoon baking powder
½ cup wheat germ
½ cup raisins
¼ cup orange juice

Yield: 32 squares

Food Exchanges: ½ starch/bread + ½ fat

Combine oil, sugar, and eggs. Beat until smooth. Add remaining ingredients and mix well. Pour into an oiled 13-by-9-inch baking pan. Bake in a 350-degree oven for 20 minutes. Cool before cutting.

Calories per square	74
Protein	2 g
Carbohydrate	9 g
Fat	4 g
Sodium	36 mg
Potassium	61 mg
Cholesterol	17 mg

Pinto Bean–Spice Cookies

½ cup sugar
½ cup vegetable oil
1 egg
1 cup mashed or puréed pinto
  beans
1 cup applesauce
1 ½ cups whole wheat flour
1 ½ teaspoons baking powder
½ teaspoon baking soda
1 teaspoon ground cinnamon
½ teaspoon ground nutmeg
¼ teaspoon ground cloves
1 cup chopped dates
¼ cup shredded coconut

Cream together sugar, oil, and egg. Add pinto beans and applesauce. Beat well. Stir in remaining ingredients, except coconut. Mix well. Pour into an oiled 13-by-9-inch baking pan. Sprinkle coconut on top. Bake in a 350-degree oven for 35 to 40 minutes.

Calories per square	112
Protein	2 g
Carbohydrate	15 g
Fat	5 g
Sodium	36 mg
Potassium	99 mg
Cholesterol	11 mg

Yield: 24 squares

Food Exchanges: 1 starch/bread
+ 1 fat

Mincemeat Cookies

1 cup mincemeat (see page 116)
½ cup vegetable oil
½ cup sugar
1 egg
1 teaspoon grated orange peel
1 teaspoon baking soda
1½ cups whole wheat flour
2 cups all-purpose flour

Beat mincemeat, oil, sugar, and egg together. Add remaining ingredients and mix well. Roll dough in small amounts onto a lightly floured board. Cut with a cookie cutter. Bake on a lightly oiled baking sheet at 350 degrees for 10 to 12 minutes.

Calories per 2 cookies	96
Protein	2 g
Carbohydrate	16 g
Fat	4 g
Sodium	32 mg
Potassium	54 mg
Cholesterol	10 mg

Yield: 60 cookies

Food Exchange: 1 starch/bread

Hamantaschen

2 cups all-purpose flour
½ cup sugar
¼ teaspoon salt
1 teaspoon orange or lemon
  rind
12 tablespoons margarine,
  room temperature
2 egg yolks
1 teaspoon vanilla extract
Sugar-free prune or apricot
  butter

Yield: 30 cookies

Food Exchanges: ½ starch/bread
+ 1 fat

Mix flour, sugar, salt, and orange rind together in a bowl. Cut in margarine until dough resembles coarse meal. Add egg yolks and vanilla. Mix just until dough sticks together. Divide dough into two parts. Wrap each in plastic and refrigerate at least 1 hour. Roll dough onto a lightly floured surface to ⅛ inch thick. Cut out 2½-inch circles with cookie cutters. Transfer circles to ungreased baking sheets. Spoon 1 teaspoon prune or apricot butter onto the center of each circle. Fold up edges of circle and shape into a 3-cornered hat by pinching corners together. Bake until golden brown, about 15 minutes.

Calories per cookie	83
Protein	1 g
Carbohydrate	8 g
Fat	5 g
Sodium	74 mg
Potassium	20 mg
Cholesterol	18 mg

Rolled Peanut Butter Cutouts

¾ *cup peanut butter*
¾ *cup sugar*
2 *eggs*
1 *teaspoon vanilla extract*
2 *cups all-purpose flour*
2 *teaspoons baking powder*
¼ *cup water*

Cream together peanut butter and sugar. Add 1 egg at a time and continue beating. Stir in vanilla, flour, and baking powder. Chill dough 3 to 4 hours or overnight for best results. Roll dough thin and cut into shapes with cookie cutters. Decorate with raisins, peanuts, and sunflower seeds.

Calories per cookie	45
Protein	1 g
Carbohydrate	6 g
Fat	2 g
Sodium	30 mg
Potassium	26 mg
Cholesterol	9 mg

Yield: 60 small cookies

Food Exchange: ½ starch/bread

Peanut Butter Cookies

½ *cup peanut butter*
¼ *cup vegetable oil*
⅓ *cup brown sugar, packed*
1 *teaspoon vanilla extract*
1 *egg*
1½ *cups all-purpose flour*
1½ *teaspoons baking powder*
½ *teaspoon baking soda*

Cream peanut butter, oil, sugar, vanilla, and egg together. Add remaining ingredients and beat well. Shape into 36 2-inch-diameter balls and place on a lightly oiled baking sheet. Flatten with a fork or the bottom of a glass. Bake in a 350-degree oven for 12 to 15 minutes, or until golden brown.

Calories per cookie	82
Protein	2 g
Carbohydrate	7 g
Fat	5 g
Sodium	67 mg
Potassium	55 mg
Cholesterol	8 mg

Yield: 36 cookies

Food Exchanges: ½ starch/bread + 1 fat

Refrigerator Spice Cookies

½ cup margarine
½ cup sugar
1 egg
1 teaspoon vanilla extract
2¼ cups all-purpose flour
½ teaspoon baking soda
1 teaspoon ground cinnamon
½ teaspoon ground nutmeg
½ cup chopped walnuts or
   pecans

Cream together margarine, sugar, egg, and vanilla. Combine flour, baking soda, cinnamon, nutmeg, and nuts in a bowl. Stir to mix. Add to creamed mixture. Beat well. Shape into 2 rolls, each 3 inches in diameter. Wrap in waxed paper and chill at least 3 hours or overnight. Cut into thin slices and bake on a lightly oiled baking sheet at 350 degrees for 10 to 12 minutes.

Yield: 72 cookies

Food Exchanges: 1 starch/bread + 1 fat

Calories per 3 cookies	108
Protein	3 g
Carbohydrate	12 g
Fat	6 g
Sodium	66 mg
Potassium	27 mg
Cholesterol	12 mg

Gingerbread Cookies

1 cup margarine
¼ cup sugar
½ cup molasses
1 egg
½ teaspoon baking soda
3½ cups all-purpose flour
1½ teaspoons ground ginger
1 teaspoon ground cinnamon

Cream together margarine, sugar, molasses, and egg. Add baking soda, flour, ginger, and cinnamon. Mix until smooth. Refrigerate for 2 hours or overnight. Roll out onto a lightly floured surface until ⅛ inch thick. Cut with a cookie cutter. Place on ungreased baking sheets. Bake in a 375-degree oven for 12 to 15 minutes.

Yield: 72 small cookies

Food Exchanges: ½ starch/bread + ½ fat

Calories per cookie	52
Protein	0
Carbohydrate	6 g
Fat	3 g
Sodium	38 mg
Potassium	41 mg
Cholesterol	4 mg

Molasses Cookies

½ cup vegetable oil
¼ cup molasses
¼ cup sugar
1 egg
2 cups whole wheat flour
2 teaspoons baking soda
1 teaspoon ground cinnamon
½ teaspoon ground ginger
¼ teaspoon ground cloves

Beat together oil, molasses, sugar, and egg. Add remaining ingredients and mix well. Chill dough for 2 hours or overnight. Form into 1-inch balls. Roll into granulated sugar and place on lightly oiled baking sheets about 2 inches apart. Bake in a 375-degree oven for 10 to 12 minutes.

Yield: 48 cookies

Food Exchange: ½ starch/bread

Calories per cookie	46
Protein	1 g
Carbohydrate	6 g
Fat	2 g
Sodium	37 mg
Potassium	45 mg
Cholesterol	6 mg

Ginger-Spice Cookies

⅓ cup vegetable oil
3 tablespoons water
1 egg
½ teaspoon vanilla extract
1 teaspoon baking powder
½ teaspoon ground cinnamon
½ teaspoon ground ginger
¼ teaspoon ground cloves
1½ cups all-purpose flour
12 packets sugar substitute
½ teaspoon ground cinnamon

Beat oil, water, egg, and vanilla together. Add baking powder, cinnamon, ginger, cloves, and flour. Stir until well blended. Roll dough onto a lightly floured surface. Cut into 2-inch rounds with a cookie cutter. Place cookies in a lightly oiled baking pan. Bake in a 375-degree oven for 7 to 10 minutes. Combine sugar substitute and cinnamon in a plastic bag or shallow dish. Place warm cookies in the bag and shake to coat with topping. Cool.

Yield: 36 cookies

Food Exchanges: ½ starch/bread + ½ fat

Calories for 2 cookies	74
Protein	1 g
Carbohydrate	8 g
Fat	4 g
Sodium	18 mg
Potassium	14 mg
Cholesterol	16 mg

Orange-Raisin Clusters

⅓ cup vegetable oil

¼ cup sugar

1 egg

2 cups whole wheat flour

2½ teaspoons baking powder

1½ teaspoons ground
  cinnamon

½ teaspoon baking soda

¼ teaspoon ground cloves

⅓ cup frozen undiluted orange
  juice concentrate

¼ cup honey

1 cup raisins

1 cup uncooked oats

¼ cup sunflower seeds

Yield: 48 cookies

Food Exchange: 1 starch/bread

Combine oil and sugar. Beat well. Add egg. Stir in flour, baking powder, cinnamon, baking soda, cloves, orange juice concentrate, and honey. When thoroughly blended, add raisins, oats, and sunflower seeds. Drop by tablespoons onto a lightly oiled baking pan. Bake in a 350-degree oven for 15 to 20 minutes or until lightly browned.

Calories per cookie	64
Protein	1 g
Carbohydrate	10 g
Fat	2 g
Sodium	29 mg
Potassium	73 mg
Cholesterol	6 mg

Sugar-free Oatmeal Cookies

1 cup whole wheat flour
1 cup oatmeal
1 teaspoon ground cinnamon
1 teaspoon baking powder
½ teaspoon baking soda
¼ teaspoon ground nutmeg
¼ teaspoon ground allspice
¼ teaspoon ground cloves
½ cup raisins
1 cup unsweetened applesauce
¼ cup water
⅓ cup vegetable oil
2 eggs
1 teaspoon vanilla extract
¼ cup finely chopped nuts

Combine all ingredients in a mixing bowl. Beat well. Drop by spoonfuls onto a lightly oiled baking sheet. Bake in a 375-degree oven for 10 to 15 minutes, or until browned.

Calories per 3 cookies	126
Protein	3 g
Carbohydrate	15 g
Fat	6 g
Sodium	66 mg
Potassium	114 mg
Cholesterol	33 mg

Yield: 48 cookies

Food Exchanges: 1 starch/bread
+ 1 fat

Carob-Oatmeal Cookies

½ cup vegetable oil
⅓ cup sugar
1 egg
⅔ cup whole wheat flour
½ cup rolled oats
¼ cup carob powder
1 teaspoon baking powder
¼ teaspoon ground cinnamon
⅛ teaspoon ground cloves
½ cup chopped walnuts or
  pecans

Yield: 24 cookies

Food Exchanges: ½ starch/bread
+ 1 fat

Cream together oil, sugar, and egg. Add flour, oats, carob powder, baking powder, cinnamon, and cloves. Beat until well blended. Stir in nuts. Drop by spoonfuls onto a lightly oiled baking pan. Bake in a 350-degree oven for 10 to 12 minutes.

Calories per cookie	89
Protein	1 g
Carbohydrate	7 g
Fat	7 g
Sodium	19 mg
Potassium	48 mg
Cholesterol	11 mg

Orange-Coconut Clusters

2 egg whites
¼ teaspoon almond extract
¼ cup sugar
1 cup toasted shredded coconut
3 tablespoons grated orange
  peel

Yield: 36 cookies

Food Exchange: ½ fruit

Beat egg whites with almond extract until soft peaks. Add sugar 1 tablespoon at a time. Beat until peaks are stiff and shiny. Fold in coconut and orange peel. Drop by teaspoons onto a baking sheet lined with waxed paper or parchment. Bake in a 350-degree oven for 10 minutes. Reduce heat to 300 degrees and bake for 15 minutes. Cool slightly before removing from paper. Store in an airtight container.

Calories per 2 cookies	30
Protein	0.5 g
Carbohydrate	4 g
Fat	1 g
Sodium	6 mg
Potassium	32 mg
Cholesterol	0

Tofu-Spice Cookies

¾ cup vegetable oil
1 cup honey
2 eggs
12 ounces tofu
2¾ cups whole wheat flour
2 teaspoons ground ginger
1 teaspoon ground cinnamon
1 teaspoon ground nutmeg
1 teaspoon baking soda
1 cup raisins
½ cup chopped walnuts
1 cup chopped dates

Yield: 48 cookies

Food Exchanges: 1 starch/bread
+ ½ fat

Combine oil, honey, eggs, and tofu in a blender, food processor, or mixing bowl. Add remaining ingredients. Mix well. Drop onto a lightly oiled baking pan. Bake in a 350-degree oven for 15 to 20 minutes.

Calories per cookie	101
Protein	2 g
Carbohydrate	14 g
Fat	5 g
Sodium	20 mg
Potassium	71 mg
Cholesterol	6 mg

Swedish Hazelnut Squares

⅓ cup margarine
⅓ cup sugar
½ teaspoon pure orange extract
1 teaspoon vanilla extract
2 eggs, separated
⅔ cup all-purpose flour
1½ teaspoons baking powder
⅔ cup coarsely ground
   hazelnuts

Yield: 36 squares

Food Exchanges: ½ starch/bread
+ 1 fat

Cream margarine and sugar together until light and fluffy. Beat in orange extract, vanilla, and egg yolks. Add flour and baking powder. Beat to blend. Spread in a lightly oiled 9-by-9-inch baking pan. Beat egg whites until stiff peaks. Fold in nuts. Spread egg white mixture over cookie dough. Bake in a 350-degree oven for 20 minutes.

Calories per 2 squares	96
Protein	2 g
Carbohydrate	8 g
Fat	6 g
Sodium	68 mg
Potassium	34 mg
Cholesterol	32 mg

10

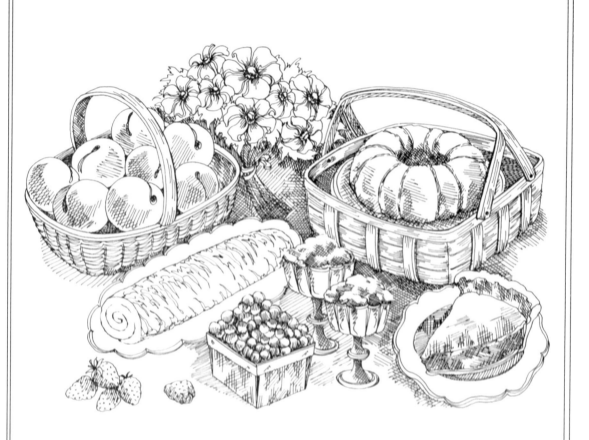

Desserts

Apple and Cheese Pizza

1 package active dry yeast
¾ cup warm water (110 degrees)
2 cups whole wheat flour
½ teaspoon ground cardamom
1 tablespoon vegetable oil
3 large apples, thinly sliced
1 cup apple juice
1 tablespoon cornstarch
½ teaspoon ground cinnamon
2 tablespoons honey
¼ cup chopped toasted pecans
1 cup grated low-fat mozzarella cheese

Yield: 10 servings

Food Exchanges: 1 lean meat + 1 starch/bread + 1 fruit + 1 fat

Dissolve yeast in warm water. Add flour and cardamom. Beat to make a soft dough. Knead in vegetable oil. Let dough rise in a warm place about 1 hour. Punch down. Press dough into a lightly greased 14-inch pizza pan. Cook apples in apple juice until tender. Drain off juice and reserve. Place apple slices on dough. Dissolve cornstarch in apple juice, cinnamon, and honey. Cook over medium heat until clear. Spread sauce over apples. Sprinkle pecans on top. Top with cheese. Bake in a 425-degree oven for 15 to 20 minutes.

Calories per serving	230
Protein	10 g
Carbohydrate	32 g
Fat	8 g
Sodium	108 mg
Potassium	224 mg
Cholesterol	13 mg

Cheesecake

1½ cups graham cracker
   crumbs
¼ cup margarine, melted
2 8-ounce packages low-fat
   cream cheese, softened
6 eggs, separated
⅓ cup sugar
1 cup plain low-fat yogurt
1½ teaspoons vanilla extract

Make crust by tossing graham crackers, and margarine together. Press into bottom of 10-inch spring-form pan. Combine cream cheese, egg yolks, and sugar in food processor or mixing bowl. Beat until smooth. Pour cream cheese mixture into bowl and stir in yogurt and vanilla. Beat egg whites until soft peaks form. Fold cheese mixture into egg whites. Pour over crust. Immediately place in preheated 400-degree oven. Reduce heat to 300 degrees and bake for 1 hour. Turn oven off and let cheesecake bake for 1 hour longer. Cool for 2 hours at room temperature before refrigerating until ready to serve.

Yield: 24 servings

Food Exchanges: ½ starch/bread
+ 2 fats

Calories per serving	142
Protein	4 g
Carbohydrate	8 g
Fat	11 g
Sodium	142 mg
Potassium	85 mg
Cholesterol	90 mg

Variation: Fold in 1 cup chocolate chips* at the same time you add the yogurt and vanilla.

Calories per serving	173
Protein	4 g
Carbohydrate	12 g
Fat	12 g
Sodium	142 mg
Potassium	85 mg
Cholesterol	90 mg

Food Exchanges: 1 starch/bread
+ 2 fats

* This recipe variation contains chocolate chips, which are high in saturated fat and sugar. Reserve this recipe variation for very special occasions only.

Frozen Fruit Delight

½ banana, sliced
24 green seedless grapes
¼ honeydew melon, cubed
¼ cantaloupe, cubed
¼ papaya, cubed (or 2 kiwis)
½ cup sliced fresh strawberries
2 tablespoons salad dressing
¼ cup plain low-fat yogurt

Yield: 6 ½-cup servings

Food Exchanges: 1 fruit + 1 fat

Combine fruit, salad dressing, and yogurt. Pack into lightly oiled loaf pan or salad mold. Freeze until firm. Defrost 5 minutes before unmolding by dipping in hot water.

Calories per serving	91
Protein	1 g
Carbohydrate	14 g
Fat	4 g
Sodium	37 mg
Potassium	306 mg
Cholesterol	3 mg

Pineapple Upside-Down Cake

8 pineapple rings or ½ cup
   pineapple chunks (packed in
   juice)
2 tablespoons molasses
⅓ cup margarine
⅓ cup honey
1 egg
1½ cups all-purpose flour
2 teaspoons baking powder
½ teaspoon baking soda
¾ cup pineapple juice
   (reserved from pineapple
   slices—add water if not
   enough juice)

Yield: 12 squares

Food Exchanges: 1 starch/bread
+ 1 fruit + 1 fat

Liberally oil 9-inch square baking pan. Arrange pineapple rings or pineapple chunks in bottom of pan. Drizzle on molasses. Beat together margarine, honey, and egg. Add rest of the ingredients. Stir until smooth. Pour batter over pineapple rings. Bake in 350-degree oven for 30 to 35 minutes. Cool.

Calories per square	180
Protein	2 g
Carbohydrate	30 g
Fat	6 g
Sodium	152 mg
Potassium	145 mg
Cholesterol	23 mg

Sufganiyot (Preserve-filled doughnuts)

2 tablespoons dry yeast
2 tablespoons sugar
¾ cup warm skim milk
2½ cups all-purpose flour
2 egg yolks
¼ teaspoon ground cinnamon
1 tablespoon soft margarine
8 teaspoons sugar-free
   strawberry preserves
Vegetable oil for frying
Sugar substitute

Dissolve yeast and sugar in milk. Add flour, egg yolks, and cinnamon. Beat well. Knead in margarine until dough is elastic. Place in an oiled bowl, cover, and let rise for 2 hours. Punch dough down. Roll dough out onto a lightly floured surface until ½ inch thick. Cut out 2-inch circles. Cover with a towel and let rise for 15 minutes. Heat oil in a frying pan. Drop doughnuts into oil and turn when brown. Drain on paper towels. Using a small spoon, fill each dough-nut with ½ teaspoon strawberry preserves. Sprinkle sugar substitute on top before serving.

Yield: 16 doughnuts

Food Exchanges: 1 starch/bread + 1 fat

Calories per doughnut	132
Protein	3 g
Carbohydrate	18 g
Fat	5 g
Sodium	29 mg
Potassium	70 mg
Cholesterol	17 mg

Fresh Fruit Ambrosia

¼ cup pineapple juice
½ cup club soda
1 banana
1 cup sliced peaches
1 cup sliced strawberries
1 cup grapes
¼ teaspoon ground cinnamon
2 tablespoons toasted wheat
   germ

Combine pineapple juice, club soda, and banana in blender. Purée until smooth. Pour over fresh fruit mixture in a bowl. Sprinkle on cinnamon. Refriger-ate until ready to serve. Sprinkle on wheat germ and serve immediately.

Yield: 6 ½-cup servings

Food Exchange: 1 fruit

Calories per serving	50
Protein	1 g
Carbohydrate	11 g
Fat	0
Sodium	2 mg
Potassium	152 mg
Cholesterol	0

Bread Pudding

2 cups (2 slices) cubed dried
  whole wheat bread
½ cup raisins
3 cups skim milk
1 tablespoon honey
2 eggs
½ teaspoon ground cinnamon
½ cup bran cereal
Ground nutmeg

Yield: 6 ½-cup servings

Food Exchanges: 1 starch/bread
+ ½ skim milk

Place bread cubes and raisins in the bottom of a lightly oiled casserole. Combine milk, honey, eggs, and cinnamon. Beat to blend. Pour over bread cubes. Sprinkle on cereal. Top with nutmeg. Bake in a 325-degree oven for 50 to 55 minutes or until a knife inserted into the center comes out clean.

Calories per ½ cup	137
Protein	8 g
Carbohydrate	23 g
Fat	3 g
Sodium	181 mg
Potassium	396 mg
Cholesterol	93 mg

Pumpkin Pudding Cake

2 cups all-purpose flour
¾ cup sugar
½ teaspoon baking soda
1 teaspoon baking powder
½ teaspoon ground cinnamon
¼ teaspoon ground cloves
1 cup cooked or canned
  pumpkin
⅓ cup vegetable oil
1 egg
½ cup raisins
½ cup chopped walnuts

Yield: 24 1-inch slices

Food Exchanges: 1 starch/bread
+ 1 fat

Combine all ingredients in a mixing bowl. Beat for 3 minutes. Pour into a 3-quart lightly oiled ring mold or a cheesecake pan. Bake in a 350-degree oven for 40 to 45 minutes. Cool for 5 minutes in the pan. Serve warm with a sprinkle of powdered sugar or a spoonful of vanilla yogurt.

Calories per slice	116
Protein	2 g
Carbohydrate	17 g
Fat	5 g
Sodium	31 mg
Potassium	70 mg
Cholesterol	11 mg

Note: This recipe contains a moderate amount of sucrose. This recipe is for occasional use only and should be carefully worked into the individual meal plan.

Sponge Roll with Strawberry Filling

4 eggs
¼ cup sugar
1 teaspoon vanilla extract
¾ cup cake flour
1 cup crème fraîche (page 114)
½ cup chopped strawberries
2 packets sugar substitute

Beat eggs, sugar, and vanilla together in a bowl with an electric mixer on high speed until mixture is thick and pale yellow, about 5 minutes. Gradually fold flour into mixture with a spatula. Spread batter evenly into a 15-by-10-inch jelly-roll pan lined with waxed paper. Bake in a 350-degree oven until golden brown, about 10 to 12 minutes. Loosen the edges from the pan and cool cake thoroughly in the pan.

Invert cake onto a towel sprinkled with powdered sugar. Remove waxed paper. Use the towel to roll up cake from the long end. Keep covered until ready to fill. Unroll cake and spread with crème fraîche mixed with strawberries and sugar substitute. Use the towel to reroll cake. Refrigerate until ready to serve. Top with sliced fresh strawberries.

Yield: 18 1-inch slices

Food Exchanges: ½ starch/bread + 1 fat

Calories per slice	87
Protein	2 g
Carbohydrate	7 g
Fat	6 g
Sodium	21 mg
Potassium	36 mg
Cholesterol	80 mg

Sponge Cake

9 eggs, separated
¾ cup sugar
2 teaspoons grated lemon peel
½ cup water
¾ cup matzo cake meal
¼ cup potato starch

Beat egg whites until stiff. Combine egg yolks, sugar, and lemon peel in a bowl. Mix until light and fluffy, about 3 minutes at medium speed with an electric mixer. Gradually add water, matzo cake meal, and potato starch. Continue beating for 2 more minutes at medium speed. Fold egg whites into batter gently but thoroughly. Pour batter into an ungreased 10-inch tube pan. Bake in a 350-degree oven about 1 hour or until cake springs back when touched with your finger. Invert the pan and cool thoroughly before removing cake from the pan.

Calories per slice	106
Protein	4 g
Carbohydrate	15 g
Fat	3 g
Sodium	39 mg
Potassium	42 mg
Cholesterol	154 mg

Yield: 24 ½-inch slices

Food Exchange: 1 starch/bread

Note: This recipe contains a moderate amount of sucrose. This recipe is for occasional use only and should be carefully worked into the individual meal plan.

Baked Apples

8 baking apples (Delicious or
   Rome Beauty)
½ cup apple juice concentrate
½ cup raisins
½ cup chopped toasted pecans
1 teaspoon ground cinnamon

Core apples and place in a baking pan. Divide concentrate among apples. Mix raisins, pecans, and cinnamon together. Spoon mixture into the center of each apple. Cover the pan with foil and bake in a 350-degree oven for 40 to 45 minutes, or until apples are tender.

Yield: 8 baked apples

Food Exchanges: 1½ fruits +
1 fat

Calories per apple	139
Protein	1 g
Carbohydrate	26 g
Fat	5 g
Sodium	2 mg
Potassium	247 mg
Cholesterol	0

Apple-Raisin Snack Cake

⅓ cup vegetable oil
2 eggs
½ cup sugar
2 cups whole wheat flour
2 teaspoons baking powder
½ teaspoon baking powder
½ teaspoon baking soda
¾ teaspoon ground cinnamon
¼ teaspoon ground nutmeg
2 cups (2 large) finely diced
   apple
½ cup raisins
¼ cup apple juice

Beat oil and eggs together. Add remaining ingredients and mix well. Pour into a lightly oiled and floured 13-by-9-inch baking pan. Bake in a 350-degree oven for 30 minutes.

Calories per slice	99
Protein	2 g
Carbohydrate	16 g
Fat	4 g
Sodium	44 mg
Potassium	82 mg
Cholesterol	23 mg

Yield: 24 1½-inch slices

Food Exchanges: 1 starch/bread
+ ½ fat

Apple Cake

2 pounds sweet apples (Golden
  Delicious)
¼ cup sugar
1 cup margarine
¼ cup honey
2 eggs
2½ cups all-purpose flour
2½ teaspoons baking powder
2 teaspoons finely grated
  orange rind
½ cup chopped walnuts

Yield: 24 1½-inch squares

Food Exchanges: 1½ starches/
breads + 2 fats

Peel and dice apples. Sprinkle sugar over them while making batter. Beat margarine, honey, and eggs until fluffy. Add flour, baking powder, orange rind, and apples. If apples do not make enough juice for a smooth batter, use ¼ cup water. Spread batter into a lightly oiled 13-by-9-inch baking pan. Sprinkle walnuts on top. Bake in a 350-degree oven for 40 to 45 minutes, or until cake tests done.

Calories per square	214
Protein	3 g
Carbohydrate	22 g
Fat	13 g
Sodium	162 mg
Potassium	64 mg
Cholesterol	30 mg

Strawberries with Blueberry Sauce

2 cups sliced fresh strawberries
½ cup fresh or frozen
  blueberries
½ teaspoon grated orange peel
⅛ teaspoon ground cinnamon
1 packet sugar substitute
4 teaspoons plain low-fat
  yogurt

Yield: 4 ⅔-cup servings

Food Exchange: 1 fruit

Divide strawberries into 4 serving dishes. Purée blueberries, orange peel, cinnamon, and sugar substitute in a blender. Pour sauce over strawberries. Top with yogurt before serving.

Calories per serving	57
Protein	1 g
Carbohydrate	9 g
Fat	0
Sodium	1 mg
Potassium	194 mg
Cholesterol	0

Poached Pears with Blueberry Sauce

3 ripe Bosc pears
2 tablespoons lemon juice
1 tablespoon grated lemon rind
1 tablespoon grated orange
  rind
6 whole cloves
1 cup blueberries
⅛ teaspoon ground cinnamon
1 packet sugar substitute

Peel pears but leave the stems attached. Rub with lemon juice. Cut each pear in half and place on plastic wrap. Sprinkle on grated lemon and orange rind. Stick 2 cloves in each pear half. Wrap plastic around pear and twist the ends together. Cook in a microwave oven on high power for 4 to 5 minutes. (To use a conventional stove, combine pear halves, lemon and orange rinds, and cloves in a saucepan with 1 cup of water—enough to cover pear halves. Poach over medium heat until pear is tender.)

Make the sauce by combining blueberries and cinnamon in a bowl. Cover tightly and microwave on high power for 2 minutes or until berries pop. (To use a saucepan, add ¼ cup water to blueberries and cook over high heat until berries pop.) Pour into a blender or food processor. Add sugar substitute and purée. Spoon sauce over pear halves in serving dishes.

Yield: 6 servings of ½ pear

Food Exchange: 1 fruit

Calories per ½ pear	63
Protein	0
Carbohydrate	16 g
Fat	0
Sodium	2 mg
Potassium	129 mg
Cholesterol	0

Peach-Oatmeal Cake

½ cup vegetable oil

¼ cup honey

1 egg

1½ cups all-purpose flour

½ cup oatmeal

1 teaspoon baking soda

2 teaspoons baking powder

½ teaspoon ground nutmeg

1 teaspoon ground cinnamon

1 cup buttermilk

2 cups (4 medium) fresh or
   frozen peach slices

Yield: 24 1½-inch squares

Food Exchanges: 1 starch/bread
+ ½ fat

Beat together oil, honey, and egg. Add remaining ingredients. Stir until smooth. Pour batter into an oiled 13-by-9-inch baking pan. Bake in a 350-degree oven for 30 to 35 minutes. Cool and cut into squares. If desired, combine 1 packet sugar substitute and ½ teaspoon ground cinnamon. Sprinkle on top of cooled cake before serving.

Calories per square	96
Protein	2 g
Carbohydrate	11 g
Fat	5 g
Sodium	74 mg
Potassium	63 mg
Cholesterol	12 mg

Fruit Leather

1 pound fresh fruit (peaches or apricots)
1 to 2 packets sugar substitute
Vegetable oil

Peel, pit, and slice fruit. Purée fruit in a food processor. Cook in a stainless steel or enamel pot over low heat until thickened, about 2 hours. Stir occasionally to prevent sticking. Remove from heat and stir in sugar substitute. Oil the bottom of a baking sheet. Pour a thin layer of thickened purée on the baking sheet. Cover with cheesecloth and allow to dry for 8 hours in the sun or for 24 hours inside. To use a conventional oven, preheat to 200 degrees. Place the baking sheet in the oven and turn off heat. Let stand for 12 hours.

Purée is ready to roll when it is dry to the touch. Cut into strips 2 to 3 inches wide. Roll up tightly and wrap in plastic to prevent drying.

Yield: 4 rolls

Food Exchange: ½ fruit

Calories per roll	37
Protein	0
Carbohydrate	9 g
Fat	0
Sodium	0
Potassium	171 mg
Cholesterol	0

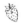

Brandied Pear Fruitcake

2 cups snipped dried pears

1½ cups (¼ pound) raisins or
   currants

¾ cup snipped dried figs

¾ cup chopped walnuts

2 cups water

⅓ cup brandy

1 tablespoon dry active yeast

¼ cup warm water

⅓ cup vegetable oil

⅓ cup sugar

¾ teaspoon ground cinnamon

3¾ to 4 cups whole wheat flour

Combine pears, raisins, figs, walnuts, 2 cups water, and brandy in a bowl. Let stand overnight or at least 3 hours. Dissolve yeast in warm water. Add oil, sugar, and cinnamon. Blend in dried fruit and nut mixture. Stir in enough flour to make a stiff dough. Beat well. Spoon dough into a 10-inch tube pan or bundt pan. Let rise in a warm place for 1 to 1 ½ hours, or until almost doubled in bulk. Bake in a 400-degree oven for 30 to 40 minutes. Cool in the pan for 10 minutes. Remove from the pan. When cooled thoroughly, wrap in foil and store at leasts 3 days before serving. Cake may be kept in an air-tight container in a cool place for several weeks before use.

Yield: 25 1-inch slices

Food Exchanges: 1 starch/bread + 1 fruit + 1 fat

Calories per slice	189
Protein	4 g
Carbohydrate	34 g
Fat	6 g
Sodium	33 mg
Potassium	253 mg
Cholesterol	0

Banana Passover Cake

6 eggs
½ cup sugar
1 cup mashed bananas
⅔ cup potato starch
¾ cup coarsely chopped
 walnuts

Separate eggs. Beat egg yolks until thick, gradually adding sugar. Stir in bananas, potato starch, and walnuts. Beat egg whites until stiff. Fold them into batter. Pour into a lightly oiled 13-by-9-inch baking pan. Bake in a 350-degree oven for 25 to 30 minutes. Serve with sliced banana and yogurt, if desired.

Calories per slice	329
Protein	8 g
Carbohydrate	44 g
Fat	15 g
Sodium	122 mg
Potassium	242 mg
Cholesterol	240 mg

Yield: 8 1-inch slices

Food Exchanges: 1 starch/bread + 1 medium-fat meat + 2 fruits + 2 fats

Note: This recipe contains more than ½ egg per serving and contains a moderate amount of sucrose. This recipe is for occasional use only and should be carefully worked into the individual meal plan.

Mincemeat Cake

¼ cup margarine, softened
1 egg
1 ½ cups mincemeat (see page 116)
½ cup apple juice
1 cup whole wheat flour
1 cup unbleached flour
1 teaspoon baking powder
½ teaspoon baking soda
½ teaspoon ground cinnamon
¼ teaspoon ground cloves
½ cup chopped nuts

Yield: 16 1-inch slices

Food Exchanges: 1 starch/bread + ½ fruit + 1 fat

Beat margarine and egg together in a bowl. Add mincemeat and apple juice. Mix well. Stir in remaining ingredients. Pour into a lightly oiled 2-quart ring mold or a tube pan. Bake in a 350-degree oven for 40 to 45 minutes. Cool for 5 minutes before removing from the pan.

Calories per slice	125
Protein	4 g
Carbohydrate	21 g
Fat	7 g
Sodium	83 mg
Potassium	132 mg
Cholesterol	21 mg

Carob-Prune Cake

⅓ cup sugar

2 tablespoons carob powder or
  cocoa

1 teaspoon ground cinnamon

½ cup vegetable oil

1 egg

¾ cup (about 25) puréed
  prunes

½ cup prune juice

1½ cups whole wheat flour

½ cup rolled oats

1 teaspoon baking powder

1 teaspoon baking soda

Yield: 24 squares

Food Exchanges: 1 starch/bread
  + 1 fat

Combine sugar, carob powder, cinnamon, oil, egg, and prunes in a bowl. Beat until smooth and creamy. Add prune juice, flour, oats, baking powder, and baking soda. Mix well. Pour batter into a lightly oiled 13-by-9-inch pan. Bake in a 350-degree oven for 25 to 35 minutes. Cool and cut into squares or bars.

Calories per square	109
Protein	2 g
Carbohydrate	15 g
Fat	5 g
Sodium	54 mg
Potassium	122 mg
Cholesterol	11 mg

Pumpkin Cheesecake

1 cup (about 20 cookies)
   crushed gingersnaps
2 tablespoons margarine
1 8-ounce package low-fat
   cream cheese, softened
1 cup low-fat ricotta cheese
1 cup skim milk plus ¼ cup
   nonfat dry milk or 1 cup
   canned evaporated skim milk
4 eggs, separated
1 cup mashed pumpkin
3 tablespoons sugar
1 teaspoon ground cinnamon
½ teaspoon ground nutmeg
¼ teaspoon ground cloves
2 tablespoons brandy or
   brandy extract

Yield: 18 1-inch slices

Food Exchanges: 1 starch/bread + 2½ fats

Make crust by combining gingersnaps and margarine in a bowl. Press mixture into the bottom of a 10-inch springform pan. Set aside. Prepare filling by beating cream cheese, ricotta cheese, milk, egg yolks, pumpkin, sugar, cinnamon, nutmeg, cloves, and brandy until light and fluffy. Beat egg whites to form soft peaks. Fold egg whites into pumpkin mixture. Pour into the pan. Bake in a 350-degree oven for 60 to 70 minutes, or until center is set. Cool on a wire rack for 1 hour before chilling.

Calories per slice	208
Protein	5 g
Carbohydrate	17 g
Fat	12 g
Sodium	149 mg
Potassium	126 mg
Cholesterol	82 mg

Note: This recipe contains more than 2 fat exchanges per serving.

Apple-Mincemeat Pie

4 cups thinly sliced baking apples, peeled
1 unbaked 9-inch pie crust
2 cups mincemeat (see page 116)
¾ cup oat bran or oatmeal
¼ cup all-purpose flour
2 tablespoons vegetable oil

Arrange apple slices in the bottom of pie crust. Spread mincemeat over apples. Combine oat bran, flour, and oil in bowl. Stir until crumbly. Sprinkle mixture on top of mincemeat. Bake in a 400-degree oven for 10 minutes. Reduce oven temperature to 375 degrees and continue baking for 25 to 30 minutes more, or until crust is golden brown. Cool.

Calories per slice	331
Protein	5 g
Carbohydrate	55 g
Fat	10 g
Sodium	111 mg
Potassium	364 mg
Cholesterol	8 mg

Yield: 10 slices

Food Exchanges: 2 starches/breads + 1½ fruits + 2 fats

Note: This recipe contains a moderate amount of sucrose. This recipe is for occasional use only and should be carefully worked into the individual meal plan.

Pumpkin-Mincemeat Pie

1 ½ cups prepared mincemeat
(see page 116)
1 9-inch pie crust
1 ½ cups canned or cooked
pumpkin
¼ cup brown sugar
1 teaspoon ground cinnamon
½ teaspoon ground ginger
1 cup skim milk
2 eggs

Spread mincemeat on the bottom of pie crust. Combine remaining ingredients in a mixing bowl and beat well. Pour pumpkin mixture over mincemeat. Bake in a 450-degree oven for 15 minutes. Reduce oven temperature to 325 degrees and continue baking for 20 to 30 minutes.

Calories per slice	212
Protein	5 g
Carbohydrate	28 g
Fat	7 g
Sodium	116 mg
Potassium	259 mg
Cholesterol	61 mg

Yield: 10 slices

Food Exchanges: 1 starch/bread + 1 fruit + 1 fat

Note: This recipe contains a moderate amount of sucrose. This recipe is for occasional use only and should be carefully worked into the individual meal plan.

Pumpkin Pie

1 16-ounce can pumpkin or 2
  cups cooked pumpkin
2 eggs
2 tablespoons honey
1 tablespoon orange juice
  concentrate
1 cup evaporated skim milk
1½ teaspoons ground
  cinnamon
½ teaspoon ground nutmeg
Dash of ground cloves
9-inch pie crust

Yield: 12 slices

Food Exchanges: 1 starch/bread
+ 1 fat

Beat pumpkin, eggs, honey, orange juice concentrate, milk, cinnamon, nutmeg, and cloves together. Pour into pie crust. Bake in a 375-degree oven for 50 to 60 minutes, or until a knife inserted into the center comes out clean.

Calories per slice	111
Protein	4 g
Carbohydrate	14 g
Fat	5 g
Sodium	106 mg
Potassium	191 mg
Cholesterol	47 mg

Nectarine Waldorf Dessert

4 (about 3 cups) apples,
  chopped
2 (about 2 cups) nectarines,
  chopped
¼ cup chopped pecans
¼ cup plain yogurt
2 tablespoons mayonnaise
1 packet sugar substitute
¼ teaspoon ground cinnamon
Nutmeg

Yield: 8 ½-cup servings

Food Exchanges: 1 fruit + 1 fat

Combine all ingredients, except nutmeg, in a mixing bowl. Toss to blend thoroughly. Chill until ready to serve. Lightly sprinkle with nutmeg just before serving.

Calories per ½ cup	105
Protein	1 g
Carbohydrate	14 g
Fat	6 g
Sodium	25 mg
Potassium	163 mg
Cholesterol	3 mg

Blueberry Torte Dessert

3 eggs, separated
1 tablespoon sugar
⅓ cup ground almonds
2½ cups fresh blueberries
2 teaspoons cornstarch
½ cup whipping cream
2 packets sugar substitute
½ cup vanilla yogurt

Beat egg yolks and sugar until light. Add almonds. Beat egg whites until stiff. Fold egg whites into egg yolk mixture. Line a 13-by-9-inch baking pan with waxed paper. Pour batter into the ban. Bake in a 325-degree oven for 12 to 15 minutes. Remove from the pan and cool. Cut into small squares.

To make blueberry sauce, purée ½ cup blueberries in a food processor or blender. Dissolve cornstarch in cream. Cook cream, remaining blueberries, and blueberry purée over low heat until thickened, about 5 minutes. Cool. Stir in sugar substitute. To serve, line a serving dish with ½ of blueberry sauce; arrange cake squares over blueberry sauce. Top with remaining sauce. Spoon on yogurt. Serve immediately.

Yield: 6 ½-cup servings

Food Exchanges: 1 skim milk + 2 fats

Calories per ½ cup	177
Protein	6 g
Carbohydrate	14 g
Fat	12 g
Sodium	357 mg
Potassium	171 mg
Cholesterol	166 mg

Blueberry Mousse

2 cups blueberries, puréed

1 teaspoon unflavored gelatin

1 egg

¼ teaspoon almond extract

3 packets sugar substitute
  (equivalent to 6 teaspoons
  sugar)

½ cup whipping cream

Combine blueberry purée and gelatin in a saucepan. Heat over very low heat just until gelatin dissolves, about 5 minutes. Remove from heat. Stir in egg and beat rapidly. Return to heat and cook just until mixture thickens, about 3 minutes. Remove from heat. Stir in almond extract and sugar substitute. Refrigerate until mixture thickens, about 1 hour. Whip cream until stiff. Fold into blueberry mixture. Chill at least 2 hours. Top with extra blueberries.

Yield: 4 ½-cup servings

Food Exchanges: 1 fruit + 2 fats

Calories per ½ cup	153
Protein	2 g
Carbohydrate	10 g
Fat	12 g
Sodium	35 mg
Potassium	118 mg
Cholesterol	111 mg

Blueberry Kugel

8 ounces (4 cups) uncooked
  fine noodles
½ cup egg substitute
2 tablespoons sugar
1½ cups low-fat cottage cheese
1 cup low-fat yogurt
¼ teaspoon salt
¼ teaspoon ground cinnamon
½ cup fresh or frozen
  blueberries
Nutmeg

Yield: 12 servings

Food Exchanges: 1 skim milk
+ ½ fruit + 1 fat

Add noodles to rapidly boiling water and cook according to directions until tender. Drain. Beat together remaining ingredients, except nutmeg. Stir in noodles. Pour into an oiled 9-inch square baking pan. Bake in a 325-degree oven for 40 to 45 minutes, or until a knife inserted into the center comes out clean. Serve warm or cold.

Calories per serving	155
Protein	8 g
Carbohydrate	18 g
Fat	6 g
Sodium	255 mg
Potassium	118 mg
Cholesterol	4 mg

Baked Apples and Mincemeat

6 small cooking apples
⅓ cup mincemeat (see page
  116)

Make a hole in the top of each apple and scoop out the core. Fill with prepared mincemeat. Place in a baking pan with ¼-inch water on the bottom. Pierce the skin of each apple with a fork in several places to keep them from cracking during baking. Bake in a 350-degree oven for about 20 minutes, or until apples are cooked thoroughly. Baking time will very greatly depending upon size and type of apples.

Calories per apple	84
Protein	1 g
Carbohydrate	20 g
Fat	1 g
Sodium	3 mg
Potassium	197 mg
Cholesterol	2 mg

Yield: 6 baked apples

Food Exchanges: 1½ fruits

Snappy Pumpkin Mousse

¼ cup water
1 package (about 1 teaspoon)
  unflavored gelatin
1 cup boiling water
1 egg
1 cup 2-percent-fat cottage
  cheese
1¼ cups canned pumpkin
3 tablespoons sugar
½ teaspoon ground cinnamon
⅛ teaspoon ground nutmeg
⅛ teaspoon ground cloves
18 gingersnaps, crushed

Pour ¼ cup cold water in a blender or food processor. Sprinkle in gelatin. Let stand for 1 minute for gelatin to soften. Add 1 cup boiling water. Cover and blend until gelatin dissolves. Add egg and cottage cheese. Purée until smooth. Combine pumpkin, sugar, cinnamon, nutmeg, and cloves in a bowl with gelatin mixture. Beat well. Pour ⅓ mixture in the bottom of an ungreased 13-by-9-inch pan. Cover with ½ crushed gingersnaps. Add another ⅓ pumpkin mixture and the remaining gingersnaps. Top with remaining pumpkin mixture. Cover and chill at least 4 hours. Unmold by dipping pan into warm water. Cut into squares to serve.

Yield: 24 1½-inch squares

Food Exchange: 1 starch/bread

Calories per square	75
Protein	3 g
Carbohydrate	10 g
Fat	3 g
Sodium	85 mg
Potassium	61 mg
Cholesterol	12 mg

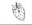
Strawberry Pretzel Delight

1 cup (about 18 whole) crushed
    pretzels
4 tablespoons melted
    margarine
1 0.3-ounce package sugar-free
    strawberry gelatin
2 cups sliced fresh strawberries

Combine pretzels and margarine. Press into a springform pan or pie pan. Bake in a 350-degree oven for 5 to 8 minutes to brown. Cool thoroughly. Meanwhile, make gelatin according to package directions using 1 cup boiling water and ¾ cup cold water. Let cool until gelatin coats a spoon. Stir in strawberries. Pour strawberry mixture into crust. Chill thoroughly, until firm, about 3 hours.

Yield: 8 slices

Food Exchanges: ½ fruit + 1 fat

Calories per slice	88
Protein	1 g
Carbohydrate	8 g
Fat	6 g
Sodium	180 mg
Potassium	74 mg
Cholesterol	0

Individual Fruitcakes

½ cup diced orange peel
½ cup diced lemon peel
½ cup golden raisins
½ cup diced dates
¼ cup brandy or orange juice
1½ cups all-purpose flour
2 teaspoons baking powder
½ teaspoon baking soda
½ teaspoon ground allspice
⅓ cup vegetable oil
2 tablespoons brown sugar
2 eggs
½ cup chopped pecans
Pineapple chunks

Combine orange peel, lemon peel, raisins, dates, and brandy in a mixing bowl. Add remaining ingredients, except pineapple. Mix well. Spoon batter into baking cups, filling each ⅔ full. Top each with pineapple chunk. Bake in a 325-degree oven for 30 to 35 minutes. Cool.

Calories per cake	212
Protein	3 g
Carbohydrate	27 g
Fat	11 g
Sodium	88 mg
Potassium	182 mg
Cholesterol	46 mg

Yield: 12 cakes

Food Exchanges: 1 starch/bread
+ 1 fruit + 2 fats

11

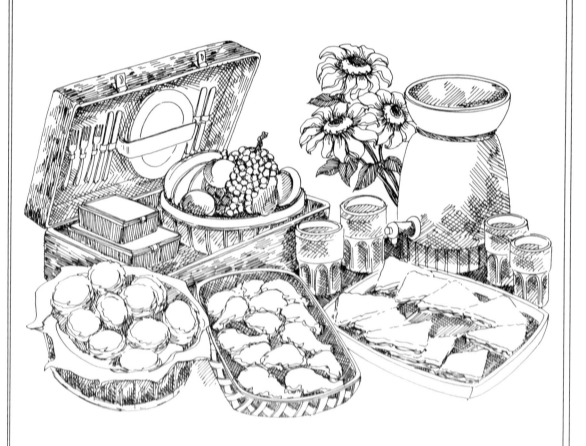

Picnic Ideas

Hearty Baked Beans

1 pound dried navy beans
1 cup chopped onion
½ cup orange juice
2 tablespoons molasses
2 tablespoons vinegar
1 teaspoon dry mustard
½ teaspoon salt
½ cup tomato sauce

Cover beans with water and let stand overnight. Drain and cover with fresh water. Cook in a covered saucepan for 1 ½ to 2 hours or until tender. Drain liquid off beans. Add remaining ingredients. Pour into a 2-quart baking dish, cover, and bake for 2 hours. Add extra tomato sauce or tomato juice, if necessary.

Yield: 12 ½-cup servings

Food Exchanges: 2 starches/breads

Calories per ½ cup	142
Protein	8 g
Carbohydrate	27 g
Fat	0
Sodium	174 mg
Potassium	525 mg
Cholesterol	0

Chili Pie

1 pound lean ground beef
1 15-ounce can kidney beans
1 onion, finely chopped
½ cup chopped green pepper
1 clove garlic, minced
1 6-ounce can tomato paste
½ cup water
1 tablespoon chili powder
6 corn tortillas
1 cup grated low-fat cheddar
  cheese

Sauté beef in a no-stick skillet until browned. Pour off fat. Mash kidney beans. Add onion, green pepper, garlic, tomato paste, water, and chili powder to ground beef. Mix well. Line a plate with tortillas. Spoon filling onto tortillas. Bake in a 350-degree oven for 25 minutes. Sprinkle on cheese. Bake for 10 minutes longer, or until cheese melts.

Yield: 6 slices

Food Exchanges: 3 lean meats + 2 starches/breads

Calories per slice	303
Protein	26 g
Carbohydrate	27 g
Fat	11 g
Sodium	273 mg
Potassium	589 mg
Cholesterol	65 mg

Shrimp-Crab-Pasta Salad

3 cups cooked sea shell pasta
1 onion, finely chopped
½ cup chopped green pepper
2 hard-cooked eggs, shelled
and chopped
1 7½-ounce can crab meat,
drained
1 7½-ounce can shrimp,
drained
½ cup diced celery
2 tablespoons minced fresh
parsley
⅛ teaspoon ground white
pepper
½ cup plain low-fat yogurt
¼ cup mayonnaise
Cherry tomatoes and cucumber
slices

Yield: 6 1-cup servings

Food Exchanges: 2 lean meats +
1 starch/bread + 1 vegetable +
1 fat

Combine pasta, onion, green pepper, eggs, crab meat, shrimp, celery, parsley, pepper, yogurt, and mayonnaise. Toss to blend. Refrigerate overnight or at least 2 hours to blend flavors. Garnish with cherry tomatoes and cucumber slices before serving.

Calories per serving	240
Protein	16 g
Carbohydrate	20 g
Fat	11 g
Sodium	101 mg
Potassium	206 mg
Cholesterol	176 mg

Brown Rice Chicken Salad

1 cup uncooked brown rice

2 cups diced cooked chicken or turkey

¼ cup chopped green pepper

2 tablespoons chopped pimento

½ cup low-calorie mayonnaise

1 tablespoon Russian dressing

1 tablespoon lemon juice

1 ripe avocado

Yield: 6 1-cup servings

Food Exchanges: 2 lean meats + 1½ starches/breads

Cook rice according to package directions. Cool. Add chicken, green pepper, pimento, mayonnaise, Russian dressing, and lemon juice. Toss to blend. Chill. Cut avocado into slices and rub with lemon juice. Arrange avocado slices around chicken salad when ready to serve.

Calories per cup	246
Protein	16 g
Carbohydrate	22 g
Fat	11 g
Sodium	289 mg
Potassium	416 mg
Cholesterol	38 mg

Eggplant Lasagna Casserole

1 pound ground turkey or
   chicken
½ cup chopped onion
¼ cup chopped green pepper
1 clove garlic, minced
1 8-ounce can tomato sauce
½ teaspoon salt
1 teaspoon dried oregano
   leaves
½ teaspoon dried basil leaves
½ teaspoon marjoram leaves
¼ teaspoon ground black
   pepper
1 pound eggplant, peeled
1 cup low-fat cottage cheese
4 ounces sliced low-fat
   mozzarella cheese

Sauté ground turkey, onion, green pepper, and garlic in a skillet. Stir in tomato sauce, salt, oregano, basil, marjoram, and pepper. Bring to a boil; reduce heat to simmer for 10 minutes. Set aside. Cut eggplant into ¼-inch-thick slices. Cook in boiling water just until tender, 2 to 3 minutes. Drain in a colander. Arrange ⅓ of eggplant slices in the bottom of an oiled baking dish. Spread ½ meat mixture over eggplant. Spoon on ½ cup cottage cheese. Lay ½ mozzarella cheese slices on top. Spoon on half the tomato sauce. Place another ⅓ eggplant slices on top of sauce. Add the remaining meat mixture, cottage cheese, and mozzarella cheese. Top with remaining eggplant slices. Spoon on rest of tomato sauce. Bake in a 350-degree oven for 40 to 45 minutes. Let stand at least 5 minutes before serving.

Yield: 4 servings

Food Exchanges: 3 lean meats +
1 starch/bread

Calories per serving	239
Protein	28 g
Carbohydrate	14 g
Fat	8 g
Sodium	363 mg
Potassium	614 mg
Cholesterol	48 mg

Lasagna

1 pound lean ground beef
1 clove garlic, crushed
1 small onion, chopped
1 8-ounce can tomato sauce
1 16-ounce can tomatoes
2 tablespoons parsley flakes
1 tablespoon dried oregano
  leaves
1 tablespoon dried basil leaves
8 ounces uncooked lasagna
  noodles
8 ounces low-fat cottage cheese
8 ounces part-skim mozzarella
  cheese
2 cups sliced zucchini

Yield: 12 servings

Food Exchanges: 3 lean meats +
1 starch/bread

Sauté beef, garlic, and onion together in a skillet. Pour off fat. Add tomato sauce, tomatoes, parsley, oregano, and basil. Simmer at least ½ hour to blend flavors. Cook lasagna noodles according to package directions. In a lightly oiled 13-by-9-inch baking dish, layer ⅓ cooked noodles, 4 ounces cottage cheese, 4 ounces mozzarella, 1 cup zucchini, and ½ meat sauce. Continue with another ⅓ cooked noodles and the remaining cottage cheese, mozzarella, zucchini, and meat sauce. Top with remaining cooked noodles. Bake in a 350-degree oven for 45 minutes. Let stand at least 10 minutes before cutting.

Calories per serving	230
Protein	21 g
Carbohydrate	22 g
Fat	7 g
Sodium	355 mg
Potassium	384 mg
Cholesterol	62 mg

Pizza Chicken

1 chicken breast, cut in half
¼ cup parmigiana sauce (see
  page 117)
¼ cup grated mozzarella
  cheese

Yield: 2 servings of ½ breast

Food Exchanges: 4 lean meats

Place chicken in a baking pan. Spread on pizza sauce and let stand in the refrigerator at least 3 hours or overnight. Bake in a 350-degree oven for 30 minutes or until tender. Sprinkle on cheese.

Calories per ½ breast	224
Protein	34 g
Carbohydrate	3 g
Fat	10 g
Sodium	299 mg
Potassium	370 mg
Cholesterol	91 mg

Impossible Pizza Pie

1 pound ground turkey sausage
   or lean Italian sausage
¼ cup grated Parmesan cheese
¼ cup chopped onion
1 clove garlic, minced
1 16-ounce can stewed
   tomatoes, drained
½ cup chopped green pepper
½ teaspoon dried basil leaves
½ teaspoon dried oregano
   leaves
2 eggs
1½ cups skim milk
¾ cup whole wheat flour
1 tablespoon baking powder
1 cup shredded part-skim
   mozzarella cheese

Yield: 6 slices

Food Exchanges: 3 lean meats +
1 starch/bread

Lightly oil a 10-inch pie plate. Cook sausage until browned; drain fat. Chop or break sausage into small pieces. Place sausage, Parmesan cheese, onion, garlic, tomato pieces, green pepper, basil, and oregano in the pie plate. Beat eggs, milk, flour, and baking powder together until smooth, about 1 minute. Pour over sausage mixture. Sprinkle on mozzarella. Bake in a 400-degree oven about 30 minutes or until a knife inserted into the center comes out clean. Cool for 5 minutes before cutting.

Calories per slice	257
Protein	24 g
Carbohydrate	18 g
Fat	10 g
Sodium	348 mg
Potassium	505 mg
Cholesterol	106 mg

Garlic and Herb Chicken

1 3-pound chicken
½ cup plain low-fat yogurt
1 tablespoon lemon juice
3 cloves garlic, minced
1 tablespoon dried oregano
leaves
1 teaspoon ground mustard
1 teaspoon paprika

Cut up chicken and remove skin. Combine yogurt, lemon juice, and garlic. Pour over chicken in a baking pan. Turn to coat chicken on all sides. Marinate at least 2 hours or overnight. Combine oregano, mustard, and paprika. Remove chicken pieces from marinade. Place on a baking sheet. Sprinkle with herb mixture. Bake in a 375-degree oven for 30 to 35 minutes, or until chicken is tender. Serve hot or cold.

Calories per serving	233
Protein	28 g
Carbohydrate	3 g
Fat	11 g
Sodium	94 mg
Potassium	306 mg
Cholesterol	87 mg

Yield: 4 3-ounce servings

Food Exchanges: 4 lean meats

Ginger-Curried Chicken Breasts

2 chicken breasts, cut in half
2 tablespoons orange juice
1 tablespoon vegetable oil
¼ teaspoon curry powder
1 tablespoon minced onion
¼ teaspoon ground ginger

Place chicken in a shallow baking dish. Combine remaining ingredients and pour over chicken. Turn to coat each piece. Cover and refrigerate at least 1 hour or overnight. Grill over medium coals for 40 to 50 minutes.

Calories per ½ breast	227
Protein	29 g
Carbohydrate	1 g
Fat	11 g
Sodium	68 mg
Potassium	262 mg
Cholesterol	83 mg

Yield: 4 servings of ½ breast

Food Exchanges: 4 lean meats

Honey-Basted Cornish Hens

2 1½-pound Cornish hens
1 tablespoon honey
2 teaspoons finely minced fresh
ginger
1 tablespoon fresh lime juice
2 teaspoons vegetable oil

Yield: 4 servings of ½ hen

Food Exchanges: 4 lean meats

Cut hens in half or leave whole. Combine honey, ginger, lime juice, and oil in a bowl. Baste hens with mixture during grilling. Grill for 20 to 35 minutes or until done.

Calories per ½ hen	269
Protein	27 g
Carbohydrate	4 g
Fat	12 g
Sodium	122 mg
Potassium	341 mg
Cholesterol	132 mg

Greek-Style Halibut Kabobs

1 pound halibut fillets
2 tablespoons vegetable oil
2 tablespoons lemon juice
1 tablespoon minced green
onion
1 small clove garlic, minced
½ teaspoon dried basil leaves
Pinch white pepper
1 green pepper, cut into
squares
10 cherry tomatoes
6 fresh mushrooms

Yield: 4 skewers

Food Exchanges: 3 lean meats +
1 vegetable + 1 fat

Cut halibut into 1½-inch chunks. Combine oil, lemon juice, onion, garlic, basil, and pepper. Add halibut chunks. Marinate overnight or at least 3 hours. Thread chunks onto 4 skewers with green pepper, tomatoes, and mushrooms. Grill 4 to 6 minutes on each side over hot coals.

Calories per skewer	229
Protein	22 g
Carbohydrate	6 g
Fat	13 g
Sodium	117 mg
Potassium	639 mg
Cholesterol	54 mg

Grilled Mullet, Basil-Style

1 pound fresh or frozen mullet
  fillets
¼ cup olive oil
1 clove garlic, minced
2 tablespoons minced fresh
  basil or 1 tablespoon dried
  basil leaves
¼ cup lemon juice

Yield: 4 fillets

Food Exchanges: 3 lean meats

Place mullet fillets on grill. Combine remaining ingredients and baste over fillets. Cook over medium coals for 5 to 7 minutes on each side. Continue basting during grilling.

Calories per fillet	200
Protein	22 g
Carbohydrate	1 g
Fat	11 g
Sodium	87 mg
Potassium	23 mg
Cholesterol	61 mg

Grilled Spicy Swordfish

¼ cup olive oil
1 teaspoon chili powder
½ teaspoon dried oregano
  leaves
¼ teaspoon dried basil leaves
2 tablespoons lemon juice
4 swordfish steaks
1 ripe avocado, peeled
1 clove garlic, peeled
¼ cup loosely packed fresh
  cilantro leaves
1 teaspoon lemon juice

Yield: 4 servings of 1 steak
with 2 tablespoons sauce

Food Exchanges: 3 lean meats +
2 fats

Combine oil, chili powder, oregano, basil, and lemon juice in a bowl. Pour over swordfish steaks in a glass dish. Turn to coat both sides. Let stand in a refrigerator for 30 minutes or overnight. When ready to prepare, grill over medium coals for 10 to 12 minutes on each side. Combine remaining ingredients in a food processor or blender. Purée until smooth. Serve avocado sauce on top of steaks.

Calories per serving	279
Protein	22 g
Carbohydrate	4 g
Fat	19 g
Sodium	115 mg
Potassium	744 mg
Cholesterol	54 mg

Lamb Burgers with Feta Cheese

1 pound ground lamb
¼ teaspoon ground cumin
½ teaspoon ground rosemary
2 ounces crumbled feta cheese
Chopped fresh cilantro or
  parsley

Divide and shape lamb into 4 patties. Sprinkle each with cumin and rosemary. Grill over hot coals for 7 to 10 minutes on each side. Top each burger with ½ ounce cheese. Keep over coals long enough for cheese to melt. Sprinkle on cilantro just before serving.

Calories per burger	196
Protein	27 g
Carbohydrate	0
Fat	9 g
Sodium	218 mg
Potassium	282 mg
Cholesterol	103 mg

Yield: 4 burgers

Food Exchanges: 4 lean meats

Pork Tenderloin à l'Orange

1 pound pork tenderloin
1 onion, thinly sliced
¼ cup orange juice concentrate

Place tenderloin on aluminum foil or parchment paper. Add onion. Pour orange juice over pork and onion. Seal edges tightly. Grill over medium coals for 30 to 40 minutes.

Calories per serving	240
Protein	25 g
Carbohydrate	9 g
Fat	11 g
Sodium	62 mg
Potassium	458 mg
Cholesterol	78 mg

Yield: 4 servings of 3 1-ounce slices

Food Exchanges: 3 lean meats + ½ fruit

Baked Fresh Pineapple

1 large ripe pineapple, peeled
1 tablespoon grated orange
  rind
½ teaspoon ground cinnamon
½ teaspoon ground nutmeg
Plain low-fat yogurt (optional)

Cut pineapple into 1-inch slices. Place slices on foil or parchment paper, and sprinkle orange rind, cinnamon, and nutmeg over slices. Wrap tightly. Grill over hot coals for 10 to 15 minutes. Top with a spoonful of yogurt just before serving, if desired.

Calories per slice	84
Protein	0
Carbohydrate	21 g
Fat	0
Sodium	2 mg
Potassium	190 mg
Cholesterol	0

Yield: 6 1-inch slices

Food Exchange: 1 fruit

Grilled Pineapple Wedges

1 large ripe pineapple, peeled
Nutmeg

Cut off the top and bottom of pineapple. Divide pineapple lengthwise into 6 wedges. Wrap each in foil and place peel side down on grill over coals. Grill for 15 minutes; unwrap and cut each wedge into bite-size pieces. Sprinkle with nutmeg.

Yield: 6 wedges

Food Exchange: 1 fruit

Bananas Grilled in the Skin

1 small ripe banana
Cinnamon

Place ripe banana on grill over hot coals. Grill for 10 minutes, turning to blacken all sides. To serve, peel off skin. Sprinkle on dash of cinnamon. Serve as a dessert or as an accompaniment to chicken.

Calories per ½ banana	53
Protein	0
Carbohydrate	14 g
Fat	0
Sodium	0
Potassium	226 mg
Cholesterol	0

Yield: 2 servings of ½ banana

Food Exchange: 1 fruit

Baked Apples on the Grill

1 apple
Cinnamon
Nutmeg

Core apple. Wrap in foil or parchment paper. Place over hot coals and grill for 10 to 15 minutes, or until a fork easily pierces skin. Serve by cutting into wedges and sprinkling on a dash of cinnamon and nutmeg.

Calories per apple	81
Protein	0
Carbohydrate	21 g
Fat	0
Sodium	1 mg
Potassium	159 mg
Cholesterol	0

Yield: 1 apple

Food Exchange: 1 fruit

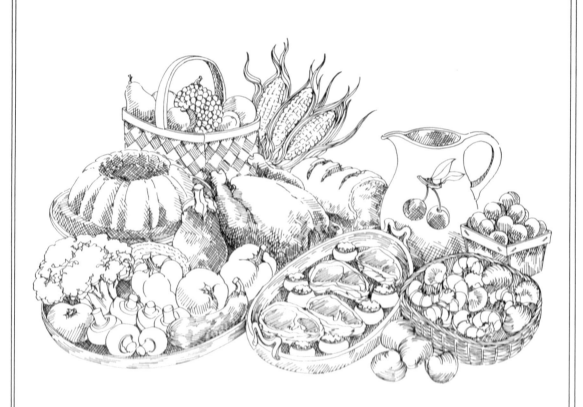

12

Exchange Lists
for Meal Planning

*T*he reason for dividing food into six different groups is that foods vary in their carbohydrate, protein, fat, and calorie contents. Each exchange list contains foods that are alike—each choice contains about the same amount of carbohydrate, protein, fat, and calories. The following chart shows the amount of these nutrients in one serving from each exchange list.

Exchange List	Carbohydrate (grams)	Protein (grams)	Fat (grams)	Calories
Starch/Bread	15	3	trace	80
Meat				
Lean	—	7	3	55
Medium-fat	—	7	5	75
High-fat	—	7	8	100
Vegetable	5	2	—	25
Fruit	15	—	—	60
Milk				
Skim	12	8	trace	90
Low-fat	12	8	5	120
Whole	12	8	8	150
Fat	—	—	5	45

As you read the exchange lists, you will notice that one choice often is a larger amount of food than another choice from the same list. Because foods are so different, each food is measured or weighed so the amount of carbohydrate, protein, fat, and calories is the same in each choice.

You will notice symbols on some foods in the exchange groups. Foods that are high in fiber (3 grams or more per exchange) are footnoted. High-fiber foods are good for you. It is important to eat more of these foods.

Foods that are high in sodium (400 milligrams or more per exchange) are footnoted; foods that have 400 milligrams or more of sodium if two or more exchanges are eaten are footnoted. It's a good idea to limit your intake of high-salt foods, especially if you have high blood pressure.

If you have a favorite food that is not included in any of these groups, ask your dietitian about it. That food can probably be worked into your meal plan, at least now and then.

The Exchange Lists for Meal Planning *are the basis of a meal-planning system designed by a committee of the American Diabetes Association and The American Dietetic Association. While designed primarily for people with diabetes and others who must follow special diets, the Exchange*

1
Starch/Bread List

Each item in this list contains approximately 15 grams of carbohydrate, 3 grams of protein, a trace of fat, and 80 calories. Whole-grain products average about 2 grams of fiber per exchange. Some foods are higher in fiber. Those foods that contain 3 or more grams of fiber per exchange are footnoted.

You can choose your starch exchanges from any of the items on this list. If you want to eat a starch food that is not on this list, the general rule is that:

- ½ cup of cereal, grain, or pasta is one exchange
- 1 ounce of a bread product is one exchange

Your dietitian can help you be more exact.

Cereals/Grains/Pasta

Bran cereals*, concentrated (such as Bran Buds®, All Bran®)	⅓ cup
Bran cereals*, flaked	½ cup
Bulgur (cooked)	½ cup
Cooked cereals	½ cup
Cornmeal (dry)	2½ Tbsp.
Grape-Nuts®	3 Tbsp.
Grits (cooked)	½ cup
Other ready-to-eat unsweetened cereals	¾ cup
Pasta (cooked)	½ cup
Puffed cereal	1½ cups
Rice, white or brown (cooked)	⅓ cup
Shredded wheat	½ cup
Wheat germ*	3 Tbsp.

* 3 grams or more of fiber per exchange.

Dried Beans/Peas/Lentils

Beans* and peas* (cooked), such as kidney, white, split, black-eyed	⅓ cup
Lentils* (cooked)	⅓ cup
Baked beans*	¼ cup

* 3 grams or more of fiber per exchange.

Starchy Vegetables

Corn*	½ cup
Corn on cob*, 6 in. long	1
Lima beans*	½ cup
Peas, green* (canned or frozen)	½ cup
Plantain*	½ cup
Potato, baked	1 small (3 oz.)
Potato, mashed	½ cup
Squash, winter* (acorn, butternut)	1 cup
Yam, sweet potato, plain	⅓ cup

* 3 grams or more of fiber per exchange.

Bread

Bagel	½ (1 oz.)
Bread sticks, crisp, 4 in. long × ½ in.	2 (⅔ oz.)
Croutons, low-fat	1 cup
English muffin	½
Frankfurter or hamburger bun	½ (1 oz.)
Pita, 6 in. across	½
Plain roll, small	1 (1 oz.)
Raisin, unfrosted	1 slice (1 oz.)
Rye, pumpernickel	1 slice (1 oz.)
Tortilla, 6 in. across	1
White (including French, Italian)	1 slice (1 oz.)
Whole-wheat	1 slice (1 oz.)

Crackers/Snacks

Animal crackers	8
Graham crackers, 2½ in. square	3
Matzoh	¾ oz.
Melba toast	5 slices
Oyster crackers	24
Popcorn (popped, no fat added)	3 cups
Pretzels	¾ oz.
Rye crisp*, 2 in. × 3½ in.	4
Saltine-type crackers	6
Whole-wheat crackers*, no fat added (crisp breads, such as Finn®, Kavli®, Wasa®)	2–4 slices (¾ oz.)

3 grams or more of fiber per exchange.

Starch Foods Prepared with Fat

(Count as 1 starch/bread exchange, plus 1 fat exchange.)

Biscuit, 2½ in. across	1
Chow mein noodles	½ cup
Corn bread, 2 in. cube	1 (2 oz.)
Cracker, round butter type	6
French fried potatoes, 2 in. to 3½ in. long	10 (1½ oz.)
Muffin, plain, small	1
Pancake, 4 in. across	2
Stuffing, bread (prepared)	¼ cup
Taco shell, 6 in. across	2
Waffle, 4½ in. square	1
Whole-wheat crackers*, fat added (such as Triscuits®)	4–6 (1 oz.)

3 grams or more of fiber per exchange.

2
Meat List

Each serving of meat and substitutes on this list contains about 7 grams of protein. The amount of fat and number of calories vary, depending on what kind of meat or substitute you choose. The list is divided into three parts based on the amount of fat and calories: lean meat, medium-fat meat, and high-fat meat. One ounce (one meat exchange) of each of these includes:

	Carbohydrate (grams)	Protein (grams)	Fat (grams)	Calories
Lean	0	7	3	55
Medium-fat	0	7	5	75
High-fat	0	7	8	100

You are encouraged to use more lean and medium-fat meat, poultry, and fish in your meal plan. This will help decrease your fat intake, which may help decrease your risk for heart disease. The items from the high-fat group are high in saturated fat, cholesterol, and calories. You should limit your choices from the high-fat group to three (3) times per week. Meat and substitutes do not contribute any fiber to your meal plan. Meats and meat substitutes that have 400 milligrams or more of sodium per exchange are footnoted. Meats and meat substitutes that have 400 milligrams or more of sodium if two or more exchanges are eaten are footnoted.

Tips

1. Bake, roast, broil, grill, or boil these foods rather than frying them with added fat.

2. Use a nonstick pan spray or a nonstick pan to brown or fry these foods.

3. Trim off visible fat before and after cooking.

4. Do not add flour, bread crumbs, coating mixes, or fat to these foods when preparing them.

5. Weigh meat after removing bones and fat, and after cooking. Three ounces of cooked meat is about equal to 4 ounces of raw meat. Some examples of meat portions are:

2 ounces meat (2 meat exchanges) =
  1 small chicken leg or thigh
  ½ cup cottage cheese or tuna
3 ounces meat (3 meat exchanges) =
  1 medium pork chop
  1 small hamburger
  ½ of a whole chicken breast
  1 unbreaded fish fillet
  cooked meat, about the size of a
    deck of cards

6. Restaurants usually serve prime cuts of meat, which are high in fat and calories.

Lean Meat and Substitutes

(One exchange is equal to any one of the following items.)

Beef:	USDA Good or Choice grades of lean beef, such as round, sirloin, and flank steak; tenderloin; and chipped beef*	1 oz.
Pork:	Lean pork, such as fresh ham; canned, cured, or boiled ham*; Canadian bacon*, tenderloin	1 oz.
Veal:	All cuts are lean except for veal cutlets (ground or cubed). Examples of lean veal are chops and roasts.	1 oz.
Poultry:	Chicken, turkey, Cornish hen (without skin)	1 oz.
Fish:	All fresh and frozen fish	1 oz.
	Crab, lobster, scallops, shrimp, clams (fresh or canned in water)	2 oz.
	Oysters	6 medium
	Tuna** (canned in water)	¼ cup
	Herring** (uncreamed or smoked)	1 oz.
	Sardines (canned)	2 medium
Wild Game:	Venison, rabbit, squirrel	1 oz.
	Pheasant, duck, goose (without skin)	1 oz.
Cheese:	Any cottage cheese**	¼ cup
	Grated Parmesan	2 Tbsp.
	Diet cheeses* (with less than 55 calories per ounce)	1 oz.
Other:	95% fat-free luncheon meat*	1½ oz.
	Egg whites	3 whites
	Egg substitutes (with less than 55 calories per ½ cup)	½ cup

* 400 milligrams or more of sodium per exchange.
** 400 milligrams or more of sodium if two or more exchanges are eaten.

Medium-Fat Meat and Substitutes
(One exchange is equal to any one of the following items.)

Beef:	Most beef products fall into this category. Examples are all ground beef, roast (rib, chuck, rump), steak (cubed, Porterhouse, T-bone), and meatloaf.	1 oz.
Pork:	Most pork products fall into this category. Examples are chops, loin roast, Boston butt, and cutlets	1 oz.
Lamb:	Most lamb products fall into this category. Examples are chops, leg, and roast.	1 oz.
Veal:	Cutlet (ground or cubed, unbreaded)	1 oz.
Poultry:	Chicken (with skin), domestic duck or goose (well drained of fat), ground turkey	1 oz.
Fish:	Tuna* (canned in oil and drained)	¼ cup
	Salmon* (canned)	¼ cup
Cheese:	Skim or part-skim milk cheeses, such as: Ricotta	¼ cup
	Mozzarella	1 oz.
	Diet cheeses** (with 56–80 calories per ounce)	1 oz.
Other:	86% fat-free luncheon meat*	1 oz.
	Egg high in cholesterol, limit to 3 per week	1
	Egg substitutes (with 56–80 calories per ¼ cup)	¼ cup
	Tofu (2½ in. × 2¾ in. × 1 in.)	4 oz.
	Liver, heart, kidney, sweetbreads (high in cholesterol)	1 oz.

* *400 milligrams or more of sodium if two or more exchanges are eaten.*
** *400 milligrams or more of sodium per exchange.*

High-Fat Meat and Substitutes

Remember, these items are high in saturated fat, cholesterol, and calories and should be used only three (3) times per week.

(One exchange is equal to any one of the following items.)

Beef:	Most USDA Prime cuts of beef, such as ribs, corned beef*	1 oz.
Pork:	Spareribs, ground pork, pork sausage** (patty or link)	1 oz.
Lamb:	Patties (ground lamb)	1 oz.
Fish:	Any fried fish product	1 oz.
Cheese:	All regular cheeses, such as American**, Blue**, cheddar*, Monterey Jack*, Swiss	1 oz.
Other:	Luncheon meat**, such as bologna, salami, pimento loaf	1 oz.
	Sausage**, such as Polish, Italian smoked	1 oz.
	Knockwurst**	1 oz.
	Bratwurst*	1 oz.
	Frankfurter** (turkey or chicken)	1 frank (10/lb.)
	Peanut butter (contains unsaturated fat)	1 Tbsp.

Count as one high-fat meat plus one fat exchange:

Frankfurter** (beef, pork, or combination)		1 frank (10/lb.)

---

* *400 milligrams or more of sodium if two or more exchanges are eaten.*
** *400 milligrams or more of sodium per exchange.*

3
Vegetable List

Each vegetable serving on this list contains about 5 grams of carbohydrate, 2 grams of protein, and 25 calories. Vegetables contain 2 to 3 grams of dietary fiber. Vegetables that contain 400 milligrams or more of sodium per exchange are footnoted.

Vegetables are a good source of vitamins and minerals. Fresh and frozen vegetables have more vitamins and less added salt. Rinsing canned vegetables will remove much of the salt.

Unless otherwise noted, the serving size for vegetables (one vegetable exchange) is:

- ½ cup of cooked vegetables or vegetable juice
- 1 cup of raw vegetables

Artichoke (½ medium)
Asparagus
Bean sprouts
Beans (green, wax, Italian)
Beets
Broccoli
Brussels sprouts
Cabbage, cooked
Carrots
Cauliflower
Eggplant
Greens (collard, mustard, turnip)
Kohlrabi
Leeks

Mushrooms, cooked
Okra
Onions
Pea pods
Peppers (green)
Rutabaga
Sauerkraut*
Spinach, cooked
Summer squash (crookneck)
Tomato (one large)
Tomato/vegetable juice*
Turnips
Water chestnuts
Zucchini, cooked

Starchy vegetables such as corn, peas, and potatoes are found on the Starch/Bread List. For free vegetables, see Free Food List on page 231.

---

400 milligrams or more of sodium per exchange.

4
Fruit List

Each item on this list contains about 15 grams of carbohydrate and 60 calories. Fresh, frozen, and dried fruits have about 2 grams of fiber per exchange. Fruits that have 3 or more grams of fiber per exchange are footnoted. Fruit juices contain very little dietary fiber.

The carbohydrate and calorie contents for a fruit exchange are based on the usual serving of the most commonly eaten fruits. Use fresh fruits or fruits frozen or canned without sugar added. Whole fruit is more filling than fruit juice and may be a better choice for those who are trying to lose weight. Unless otherwise noted, the serving size for one fruit exchange is:

- ½ cup of fresh fruit or fruit juice
- ¼ cup of dried fruit

Fresh, Frozen, and Unsweetened Canned Fruit

Apple (raw, 2 in. across)	1 apple
Applesauce (unsweetened)	½ cup
Apricots (medium or raw)	4 apricots
Apricots (canned)	½ cup, or 4 halves
Banana (9 in. long)	½ banana
Blackberries* (raw)	¾ cup
Blueberries* (raw)	¾ cup
Cantaloupe (5 in. across)	⅓ melon
(cubes)	1 cup
Cherries (large, raw)	12 cherries
Cherries (canned)	½ cup
Figs (raw, 2 in. across)	2 figs
Fruit cocktail (canned)	½ cup
Grapefruit (medium)	½ grapefruit
Grapefruit (segments)	¾ cup
Grapes (small)	15 grapes
Honeydew melon	
(medium)	⅛ melon
(cubes)	1 cup
Kiwi (large)	1 kiwi
Mandarin oranges	¾ cup
Mango (small)	½ mango
Nectarine* (2½ in. across)	1 nectarine
Orange (2½ in. across)	1 orange
Papaya	1 cup
Peach (2¾ in. across)	1 peach, or ¾ cup
Peaches (canned)	½ cup, or 2 halves
Pear	½ large, or 1 small
Pears (canned)	½ cup, or 2 halves

* *3 grams or more of fiber per exchange.*

Persimmon (medium, native)	2 persimmons
Pineapple (raw)	¾ cup
Pineapple (canned)	⅓ cup
Plum (raw, 2 in. across)	2 plums
Pomegranate*	½ pomegranate
Raspberries* (raw)	1 cup
Strawberries* (raw, whole)	1¼ cups
Tangerine* (2½ in. across)	2 tangerines
Watermelon (cubes)	1¼ cups

* 3 grams or more of fiber per exchange.

Dates	2½ medium
Figs*	1½
Prunes*	3 medium
Raisins	2 Tbsp.

* 3 grams or more of fiber per exchange.

Fruit Juice

Apple juice/cider	½ cup
Cranberry juice cocktail	⅓ cup
Grape juice	⅓ cup
Grapefruit juice	½ cup
Orange juice	½ cup
Pineapple juice	½ cup
Prune juice	⅓ cup

Dried Fruit

| Apples* | 4 rings |
| Apricots* | 7 halves |

5
Milk List

Each serving of milk or milk products on this list contains about 12 grams of carbohydrate and 8 grams of protein. The amount of fat in milk is measured in percent (%) of butterfat. The calories vary, depending on what kind of milk you choose. The list is divided into three parts based on the amount of fat and calories: skim/very low-fat milk, low-fat milk, and whole milk. One serving (one milk exchange) of each of these includes:

	Carbohydrate (grams)	Protein (grams)	Fat (grams)	Calories
Skim/Very Low-fat	12	8	trace	90
Low-fat	12	8	5	120
Whole	12	8	8	150

Milk is the body's main source of calcium, the mineral needed for growth and repair of bones. Yogurt is also a good source of calcium. Yogurt and many dry or powdered milk products have different amounts of fat. If you have questions about a particular item, read the label to find out the fat and calorie content.

Milk is good to drink, but it can also be added to cereal, and to other foods. Many tasty dishes, such as sugar-free pudding, are made with milk (see the Combination Foods List on page 232). Add life to plain yogurt by adding one of your fruit exchanges to it.

Skim and Very Low-fat Milk

Skim milk	1 cup
½% milk	1 cup
1% milk	1 cup
Low-fat buttermilk	1 cup
Evaporated skim milk	½ cup
Dry nonfat milk	⅓ cup
Plain nonfat yogurt	8 oz.

Low-fat Milk

2% milk	1 cup
Plain low-fat yogurt (with added nonfat milk solids)	8 oz.

Whole Milk

The whole milk group has much more fat per serving than the skim and low-fat groups. Whole milk has more than 3¼% butterfat. Try to limit your choices from the whole milk group as much as possible.

Whole milk	1 cup
Evaporated whole milk	½ cup
Whole plain yogurt	8 oz.

6
Fat List

Each serving on the fat list contains about 5 grams of fat and 45 calories.

The foods on the fat list contain mostly fat, although some items may also contain a small amount of protein. All fats are high in calories and should be carefully measured. Everyone should modify fat intake by eating unsaturated fats instead of saturated fats. The sodium content of these foods varies widely. Check the label for sodium information.

Unsaturated Fats

Avocado	⅛ medium	Pecans	2 whole
Margarine	1 tsp.	Peanuts	20 small
Margarine*, diet	1 Tbsp.		or 10 large
Mayonnaise	1 tsp.	Walnuts	2 whole
Mayonnaise*, reduced-calorie	1 Tbsp	Other nuts	1 Tbsp.
		Seeds, pine nuts, sunflower (without shells)	1 Tbsp.
Nuts and Seeds:			
Almonds, dry roasted	6 whole		
Cashews, dry roasted	1 Tbsp.	Pumpkin seeds	2 tsp.

* 400 milligrams or more of sodium if two or more exchanges are eaten.

		Saturated Fats	
Oil (corn, cottonseed, safflower, soybean, sunflower, olive, peanut)	1 tsp.		
		Bacon*	1 slice
		Butter	1 tsp.
Olives*	10 small or 5 large	Chitterlings	½ ounce
		Coconut, shredded	2 Tbsp.
		Coffee whitener, liquid	2 Tbsp.
Salad dressing, mayonnaise-type	2 tsp.	Coffee whitener, powder	4 tsp.
		Cream (light, coffee, table)	2 Tbsp.
Salad dressing, mayonnaise-type, reduced-calorie	1 Tbsp.	Cream (heavy, whipping)	1 Tbsp.
		Cream, sour	2 Tbsp.
Salad dressing* (oil varieties)	1 Tbsp.	Cream cheese	1 Tbsp.
		Salt pork*	¼ ounce
Salad dressing**, reduced-calorie	2 Tbsp.		

* 400 milligrams or more of sodium if two or more exchanges are eaten.
** 400 milligrams or more of sodium per exchange.

Free Foods

A free food is any food or drink that contains less than 20 calories per serving. You can eat as much as you want of those items that have no serving size specified. You may eat two or three servings per day of those items that have a specific serving size. Be sure to spread them out through the day.

Drinks:
Bouillon* or broth without fat
Bouillon, low-sodium
Carbonated drinks, sugar-free

Carbonated water
Club soda
Cocoa powder, unsweetened (1 Tbsp.)

Coffee / Tea
Drink mixes, sugar-free
Tonic water, sugar-free

* 400 milligrams or more of sodium per exchange.

FREE FOODS (cont.)

Nonstick pan spray

Fruit
Cranberries,
  unsweetened
  (½ cup)
Rhubarb, unsweetened
  (½ cup)

Vegetables
  (*raw, 1 cup*)
Cabbage
Celery
Chinese cabbage*
Cucumber
Green onion
Hot peppers
Mushrooms

Radishes
Zucchini*

Salad greens
Endive
Escarole
Lettuce
Romaine
Spinach

Sweet Substitutes
Candy, hard, sugar-free
Gelatin, sugar-free
Gum, sugar-free
Jam / Jelly, sugar-free
  (less than 20 cal./2
  tsp.)

Pancake syrup, sugar-free
  (1–2 Tbsp.)
Sugar substitutes
  (saccharin, aspartame)
Whipped topping
  (2 Tbsp.)

Condiments
Catsup (1 Tbsp.
Horseradish
Mustard
Pickles**, dill,
  unsweetened
Salad dressing,
  low-calorie (2 Tbsp.)
Taco sauce (3 Tbsp.)
Vinegar

---

* 3 grams or more of fiber per exchange.
** 400 milligrams or more of sodium per exchange.

Seasonings can be very helpful in making food taste better. Be careful of how much sodium you use. Read the label, and choose those seasonings that do not contain sodium or salt.

Basil (fresh)
Celery seeds
Chili powder
Chives
Cinnamon
Curry
Dill
Flavoring extracts
  (vanilla, almond,
  walnut, peppermint,
  butter, lemon, etc.)

Garlic
Garlic powder
Herbs
Hot pepper sauce
Lemon
Lemon juice
Lemon pepper
Lime
Lime juice
Mint
Onion powder
Oregano

Paprika
Pepper
Pimento
Soy sauce*
Soy sauce*, low-sodium
  ("lite")
Spices
Wine, used in cooking
  (¼ cup)
Worcestershire sauce

---

* 400 milligrams or more of sodium per exchange.

Combination Foods

Much of the food we eat is mixed together in various combinations. These combination foods do not fit into only one exchange list. It can be quite hard to tell what is in a certain casserole or baked food item. This is a list of average values for some typical combination foods. This list will help you fit these foods into your meal plan. Ask your dietitian for information about any other foods you'd like to eat. The *American Diabetes Association/ American Dietetic Association Family Cookbooks* and the *American Diabetes Association Holiday Cookbook* have many recipes and further information about many foods, including combination foods. Check your library or local bookstore.

Food	Amount	Exchanges
Casseroles, homemade	1 cup (8 oz.)	2 starch, 2 medium-fat meat, 1 fat
Cheese pizza*, thin crust	¼ of 15 oz. or ¼ of 10″	2 starch, 1 medium-fat meat, 1 fat
Chili with beans* ** (commercial)	1 cup (8 oz.)	2 starch, 2 medium-fat meat, 2 fat
Chow mein* (without noodles or rice)	2 cups (16 oz.)	1 starch, 2 vegetable, 2 lean meat
Macaroni and cheese*	1 cup (8 oz.)	2 starch, 1 medium-fat meat, 2 fat
Soup		
Bean* **	1 cup (8 oz.)	1 starch, 1 vegetable, 1 lean meat
Chunky, all varieties*	10 ¾ oz. can	1 starch, 1 vegetable, 1 medium-fat meat
Cream* (made with water)	1 cup (8 oz.)	1 starch, 1 fat
Vegetable* or broth-type*	1 cup (8 oz.)	1 starch
Spaghetti and meatballs* (canned)	1 cup (8 oz.)	2 starch, 1 medium-fat meat, 1 fat
Sugar-free pudding (made with skim milk)	½ cup	1 starch
If beans are used as a meat substitute		
Dried beans**, peas**, lentils**	1 cup (cooked)	2 starch, 1 lean meat

* 400 milligrams or more of sodium per exchange.
** 3 grams or more of fiber per exchange.

Foods for Occasional Use

Moderate amounts of some foods can be used in your meal plan, in spite of their sugar or fat content, as long as you can maintain blood-glucose control. The following list includes average exchange values for some of these foods. Because they are concentrated sources of carbohydrate, you will notice that the portion sizes are very small. Check with your dietitian for advice on how often and when you can eat them.

Food	Amount	Exchanges
Angel food cake	1/12 cake	2 starch
Cake, no icing	1/12 cake, or a 3" square	2 starch, 2 fat
Cookies	2 small (1¾" across)	1 starch, 1 fat
Frozen fruit yogurt	1/3 cup	1 starch
Gingersnaps	3	1 starch
Granola	¼ cup	1 starch, 1 fat
Granola bars	1 small	1 starch, 1 fat
Ice cream, any flavor	½ cup	1 starch, 2 fat
Ice milk, any flavor	½ cup	1 starch, 1 fat
Sherbet, any flavor	¼ cup	1 starch
Snack chips*, all varieties	1 oz.	1 starch, 2 fat
Vanilla wafers	6 small	1 starch

* 400 milligrams or more of sodium if two or more exchanges are eaten.

Index

A Note About the Authors

The American Diabetes Association is the nation's largest voluntary health organization dedicated to preventing and curing diabetes and to improving the lives of all people affected by diabetes.

Betty Wedman is manager of Clinical Nutrition at St. Anthony's Hospital in St. Petersburg, Florida. She holds professional memberships in The American Dietetic Association, the American Association of Diabetes Educators, and the American Diabetes Association. As past president of the American Association of Diabetes Educators, Ms. Wedman has traveled throughout the world sharing her diabetes education techniques.